THE MENTAL HEALTH OF WOMEN

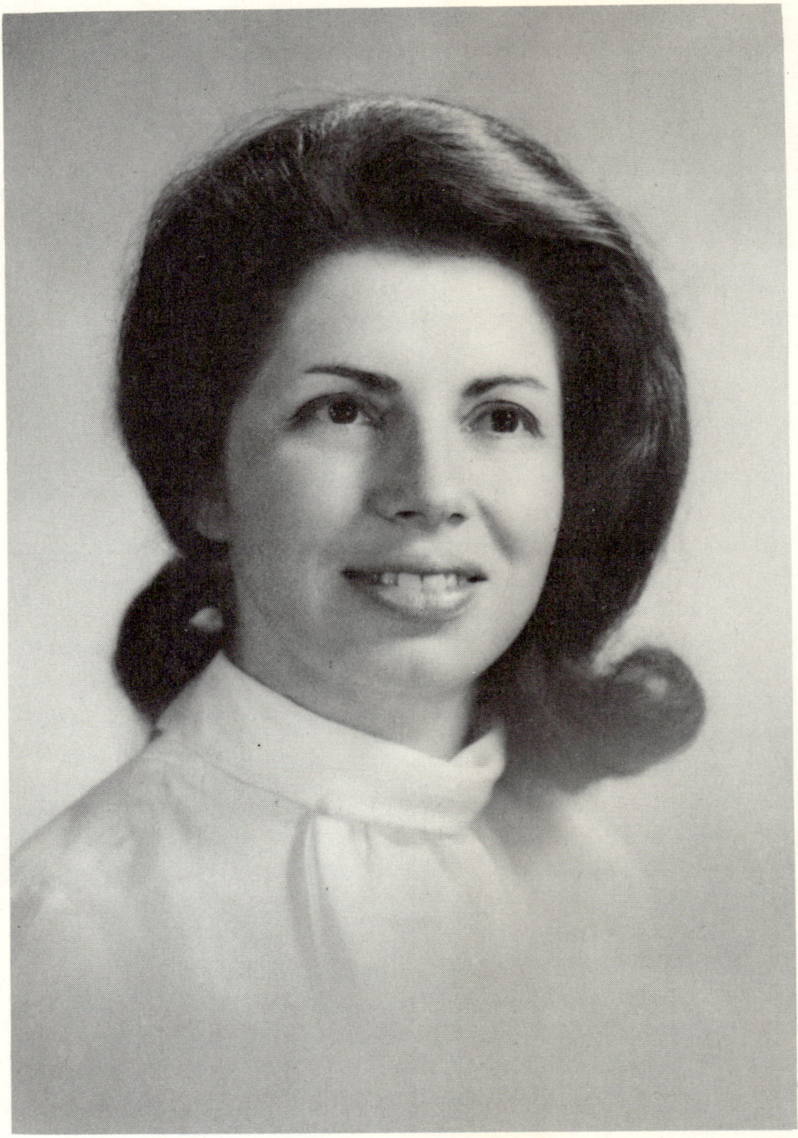

Marcia Guttentag

THE MENTAL HEALTH OF WOMEN

Edited by

Marcia Guttentag

Graduate School of Education
Harvard University
Cambridge, Massachusettes

Susan Salasin

Mental Health Services
Development Branch
National Institute of Mental Health
Rockville, Maryland

Deborah Belle

Graduate School of Education
Harvard University
Cambridge, Massachusetts

1980

ACADEMIC PRESS

A Subsidiary of Harcourt Brace Jovanovich, Publishers

New York London Toronto Sydney San Francisco

This is a volume in

PERSONALITY AND PSYCHOPATHOLOGY

A complete list of titles in this series appears at the end of this volume.

The views presented in this book are those of the editors and the authors and do not necessarily reflect the views of the National Institute of Mental Health or the United States Government.

ACADEMIC PRESS, INC.
111 Fifth Avenue, New York, New York 10003

United Kingdom Edition published by
ACADEMIC PRESS, INC. (LONDON) LTD.
24/28 Oval Road, London NW1 7DX

Library of Congress Cataloging in Publication Data
Main entry under title:

The Mental health of women.

(Personality and psychopathology series)
Includes bibliographies.
1. Women--Mental health. 2. Sex differences (Psychology) 3. Depression, Mental. I. Guttentag, Marcia. II. Salasin, Susan. III. Belle, Deborah. [DNLM: 1. Depression. 2. Mental disorders--Mental health services--Utilization--United States. 3. Sex factors. 4. Women. W1 PE861 / WM100 M54983]
RC451.4.W6M46 362.2'042 79-8543
ISBN 0-12-310850-0

PRINTED IN THE UNITED STATES OF AMERICA

80 81 82 83 9 8 7 6 5 4 3 2 1

In Tribute

A Personal Remembrance of a Special Friend

Marcia—The essence of her life as I knew her was to encourage and inspire others to maximize the use of opportunities. Marcia said of my husband, Senator Harrison Williams, Jr., "You serve as a model of selfless dedication for all of us." My husband and I share the same sentiment about Marcia's enormous influence on our lives.

I am attempting to write with my heart and mind filled with all of the beautiful memories of someone special!

It is impossible to write adequately of what Marcia meant to all of us. She was life—spontaneous, happy, eager, anxious to know the difficulty, and eager to ease the burden. How many times I would call Marcia when we had difficult legislation and describe what was happening, and how instant the response was. In a more personal way, it is impossible to write adequately of her because of her aid and comfort, her understanding, her ability to right the wrongs inflicted on people, her courage to fight lonely battles to encourage maximum opportunity for all peoples.

The legacy Marcia leaves us is incorporated in the important issues expressed in her work and in this book, and is much like the dedication in Will Durant's The Story of Philosophy:

> Grow strong, my comrade . . . . That you may stand unshaken when I fall; that I may know the shattered fragments of my song will come at last to finer melody in you; That I may tell my heart that you begin where passing I leave off, and fathom more."

In tribute to Marcia, I would like to pay respect to the importance that her work has for the legislative initiatives underway in the Congress that so affect the lives of women and their children.

JEANETTE WILLIAMS

CONTENTS

LIST OF CONTRIBUTORS

Numbers in parentheses indicate the pages on which the authors' contributions begin.

James W. Baxter (129), Program Evaluation Resource Center, Minneapolis, Minnesota 55415

Deborah Belle (1, 21, 155), Harvard University, Graduate School of Education, Appian Way, Cambridge, Massachusetts 02138

Noreen Goldman (21, 31), Office of Population Research, Princeton University, Princeton, New Jersey 08540

Thomas J. Kiresuk (129), Program Evaluation Resource Center, Minneapolis, Minnesota 55415

Gerald L. Klerman (57), Administrator, ADAMHA, Parklawn Building, Rockville, Maryland 20857

Vivian Parker Makosky (111), Department of Psychology, Saint Lawrence University, Canton, New York 13617

Lenore Sawyer Radloff (93), Center for Epidemiologic Studies and Division of Biometry and Epidemiology, National Institute of Mental Health, Rockville, Maryland 20857

Renee Ravid (31), 200 Pinehurst Avenue, New York, New York 10033

Susan Salasin (155), Mental Health Services, Development Branch, National Institute of Mental Health, Rockville, Maryland 20205

Susan K. Schultz (129), Program Evaluation Resource Center and the School of Social Work, The University of Minnesota, Minneapolis, Minnesota 55415

Myrna M. Weissman (57), Yale University School of Medicine, Department, of Psychology & Epidemiology, Depression Research Unit, Connecticut Mental Health Center, New Haven, Connecticut 06510

FOREWORD: STUDIES ON MENTAL ILLNESS

So new is the women's movement and so old are the burdens that society thrusts on our sex, that we are all pioneers in the world of women, all guinea pigs in our personal world.

Therefore, it was inevitable that two forces should come together: the women's movement and the women who are mentally ill. It took 200 years to happen. Until 1975, no study had been undertaken to see why so many women—the ignored sex, the shadow citizens—were suffering high rates of mental illness. Who was this rising statistic and why?

Then, suddenly, there she was under the microscopes and on the charts of researchers at Harvard and the National Institute of Mental Health. Strange that it should take so long to begin when it was so obviously essential to the well-being of half the population. But it did begin on a day in 1975 when an impassioned Harvard psychologist, Dr. Marcia Guttentag, who knew the trauma of raising young children alone and Susan Salasin, the innovative mental health services expert who had experienced victimization, became convinced that perhaps women were mentally sick because society made them sick, because each day the life conditions they were forced to endure demanded more of them, in breadwinning and child caring and offered only powerlessness in return. It would get worse as women's lives became more complex and diverse, more demanding.

So the studies in this book were telescoped to bring focus on hundreds of studies around the world of thousands of women with all sorts of life conditions.

And what came out was a medical fact: Women are the more depressed sex, but women struggle to do more about it. Are they doomed to struggle forever? What came out was that the most depressed of all are the low-income women from age 25 to 45, the women who live each day in a world in which welfare is the tyrant as well as the salvation. This will be the next frontier and before the ink is dry on this book, the Family and Stress Project will be under way. There will be other women in future stress studies. To understand mental illness—depression and the more serious forms—we must understand the way women live and how this can be changed to lessen stress.

For years to come, the pain of women in stress will be lessened because of Marcia Guttentag and Susan Salasin. For me they embody the words of Gloria Steinem: "I have met brave women who are exploring the outer edge of human possibility with no history to guide them and with a courage to make themselves vulnerable in a way that I find moving beyond words."

LIZ CARPENTER
Co-chair, ERAmerica

PREFACE

In a collaborative research effort, co-sponsored by Harvard University and the NIMH, answers were sought to one broad question: What is the state of mental health of women in this country, and how does it differ, if at all, from the mental health of men? The troubling picture that emerges is of the very high rates of depression in women, particularly low-income women with young children. Both sexes utilize mental health facilities at equal rates, but the leading diagnosis for men is alcoholism, whereas for women it is depression. This book is about depression in women.

What is unique about *The Mental Health of Women* is the combination of hard data on women's experience of mental health problems, theoretical analysis of the significance of women's patterns of mental illness, and concrete discussion of practice and policy issues.

The data on women's mental health are authoritative. They come from the several most important types of treatment facilities, not just from one type of treatment facility. Because no type of treatment facility is representative of all types, this is crucial. No other work before has brought together data from these several types of treatment facilities. The data are also carefully age-adjusted so that age effects do not swamp or disguise sex differences or similarities. Not only are there data on treated mental health problems, but there are also data on untreated mental health problems.

The book emphasizes depression, and it includes the thinking of some of the nations's top experts on depression in women (Weissman, Klerman, and Radloff). But it is not limited to a single perspective. The chapter by

Klerman and Weissman considers all of the important current theories on depression in women. Additional attention is given to the stress theory with a separate chapter devoted to women's experience of stress (and the attempts to measure stress).

In a time of rapidly changing notions about appropriate therapy for women, Kiresuk, Schultz, and Baxter's chapter has practical suggestions for evaluating the usefulness of therapy. The Prologue by Williams puts mental health issues in the larger political and social context in which they are, in fact, embedded.

It is with inexpressible sadness that, just as these findings developed, we experienced the sudden death of Marcia Guttentag of a heart attack at age 45. We feel that her spirit still guides us, however, particularly in the ongoing research in which we are investigating the reasons why low-income mothers have the highest rate of depression of any demographic group, and developing a plan of action to protect women and children against this epidemic of depression. This whole body of work stands as a tribute to what Marcia Guttentag hoped to accomplish for women.

In memoriam, all royalties from this book will go to Marcia's children.

ACKNOWLEDGMENTS

This book is an outgrowth of the Women and Mental Health Services Project. The initial goals of the project were to discover and examine sex differences in mental health and to pinpoint types of people of both sexes who are at risk for mental health problems. The basic data and many of the analyses used in this work were obtained from the Biometry Branch of the National Institute of Mental Health. We want to thank Morton Kramer, Carl Taube, and Paul Henderson for their helpful suggestions in this work and for their generosity in making all of the National Institute of Mental Health statistical data available to us. Within the Women and Mental Health Services Project, Wendy Willson Legge planned and coordinated the analysis of data.

No thanks are adequate to convey the extraordinary contributions to this research effort by the National Advisory Committee, chaired by Jeanette Williams. Very special contributors to the earlier phases of this effort have been Liz Carpenter, Frances Lear, Libby Cater, and Amitai Etzioni. In addition, Paul Weiss has made sustained and outstanding philosophical contributions as to how to think about the issues in this book.

Our deepest thanks are due to Howard Davis, chief of the Mental Health Services Development Branch at the National Institute of Mental Health. It is because of his long-standing commitment to fostering better mental health services for all people that the idea for the project was generated in the wake of the momentum of the women's movement and made this effort possible.

PROLOGUE: PUBLIC POLICY AND WOMEN

In just a few decades we have seen some very important changes—sometimes startling changes—in the nation and the world. Consider for a moment how television, superhighways, computers, plastics, wonder drugs, food processing, freezers, and jet planes have changed the face of America and the way Americans live—and all of this in the last 30 years! All this rapid change has been accompanied by a record of progress and improvement in the quality of life for most people in this country.

Unfortunately, however, there have been times when we have excluded some people from participating in our Nation's growth. For the first hundred years we excluded blacks. We used them as slaves to shoulder many of our burdens, but gave them little chance for anything more. It took a civil war and another hundred years before we began to move away from that unhappy record. In various ways and at various times, the same treatment we gave to blacks has been accorded to Jews, Puerto Ricans, American Indians, and numerous other cultural and ethnic groups in this country. In sum, we have too often overlooked the fact that each one of us is a living human being with something very special to contribute to the progress of our society.

More recently, we have come to recognize that we have accorded that same kind of poor treatment to women in our society. For too long a women's place was viewed as in the kitchen, raising children, and cleaning her husband's house. And to earn an extra dollar to make ends meet we allowed women to work in the sweatshops of the garment factories or as waitresses or salesgirls.

But during World War II the role of women began to change—dramatically. Women received the opportunity to serve in professional capacities in federal, state, and local government—as well as in clerical jobs. Women became doctors and lawyers as well as nurses and legal stenographers. Women taught in colleges and universities as well as in grammar schools.

That was the beginning.

It was then that women—and even some men—realized that in the past their opportunities had been severely restricted. No longer could we be complacent and say that women should have the same opportunities as men *only* when there were no men available to take advantage of those opportunities. The changing role for women would have to bring a change in our whole way of doing things. All of our values and attitudes would have to be changed—not just the values and attitudes of men, but of women too!

Clearly then we as a nation have been and are still in the throes of major upheaval with respect to changing sex roles. And as has always been the case, this important social change has had a profound impact on public policy which has been further translated into legislation.

It is this legislative activity which has been necessary to bring a sense of security, well-being, and stability to women, men, and their children and families as they attempt to cope with changing patterns of behavior and activities between the sexes. In a very real sense it is this legislative activity which has served to codify a basic framework of rights and opportunities which not only further the goal of sexual equality in itself, but also help to strengthen the mental health of the people as we adjust to a changing society.

There have been a variety of legislative efforts which are designed to deal with these problems and issues. In the more than 20 years I have been working in the Congress, perhaps the most significant initiatives have been with respect to participation of women in the work force. As more and more women—both married and single—entered the work force, it became clear that they were not receiving adequate and equal pay. This became a particularly acute problem as women were gaining more responsible positions with greater decision-making roles. In 1963 the Congress finally responded to this greatest of injustices by enacting the Equal Pay Act. The importance of this law went far beyond the correction of basic inequity of lower pay for substantially equal work. Indeed, this law, by ensuring the right of equal pay, helped overcome a major factor which produced and underscored psychological inferiority and mental stress in female workers. Thus, we have a first and paramount example of legislation which served the dual purpose of correcting a societal injustice while at the same time helping to improve the mental health of the nation's women.

But this is not all.

Nine years after the Equal Pay Act, it became clear that the need existed to ensure that women were provided the same protections as minority groups in the enforcement of our equal employment opportunity law. Thus, in 1972 under the leadership of Senator Harrison Williams, Chairman of the Senate Human Resources Committee, the Congress passed amendments to Title VII of the Civil Rights Act. Perhaps the most significant of these amendments was the provision that added sex discrimination to the list of prohibited employment activities. And later, in 1974, the addition of domestic workers to those covered by the minimum wage law became a reality.

All of these efforts are examples of what can be done in the public policy sphere with quite positive effects on the personal, and consequently mental, well-being of women. The financial independence, which accrues to women as a result of more equal opportunities in the job market, is clearly a major factor that will enhance their self-respect and self-worth. And along with this comes the emotional freedom and other similar, positive mental attitudes that are developed and reinforced as a result of living more completely up to one's potential as a total human being. Yes, the freedom from routine physical tasks of housework so as to be able to develop better academic and social skills necessary for success in the working world is bound to enhance anyone's self-image and, therefore, a woman's mental health.

It is important to remember, as women become an even greater part of our work force in each strata of every profession, their needs will undoubtedly change. Stress from the work environment or workplace setting will assuredly affect the health needs and services that will be needed by women in the future. Support systems in communities will need to respond to the physical and mental needs of working women.

It is clear then that the mental health of women in our changing society can be directly affected by the way we translate public policy trends into legislation. These are truly complex issues, but they are responded to by the legislative branch in a very sophisticated fashion. The Congress is filled with the capability of meeting both immediate and future needs all at the same time. It is an organization that must be used more often with the creativity and breadth that are so important to us as a people. Thus, we must continue to have the confidence that the legislative process will continue to play a leading role in both the fashioning of public policy and, as such, in compassionately responding to the basic human needs of the totality of our society.

JEANETTE S. WILLIAMS
U.S. Senate Committee on Labor and Human Resources

THE MENTAL HEALTH OF WOMEN

Chapter 1

WHO USES MENTAL HEALTH FACILITIES?

Deborah Belle

Every year many Americans enter mental hospitals and use outpatient psychiatric services. Such experiences are far more common, however, within certain portions of the population. Men and women who are separated or divorced, women who head families, children in female-headed families, nonwhite men—all are overrepresented in mental health facilities in relation to their proportions in the population. Although use of mental health services is not an absolute indication of mental illness, high rates of treatment among these groups are signs of a population "at risk."

The Women and Mental Health Services Project, directed by Marcia Guttentag of Harvard University and Susan Salasin of the National Institute of Mental Health, examined sex differences in patterns of utilization of and treatment in mental health facilities and of diagnoses made to pinpoint types of people who are most likely to have contact with such facilities. The Project analyzed the most recent data available, generally from 1969 to 1973. The data were obtained from state and county mental hospitals, community mental health centers, outpatient psychiatric services, general hospital inpatient psychiatric units, private mental hospitals, and children's facilities.

The basic data and many of the analyses used in the report were obtained from the Biometry branch of the National Institute of Mental Health; analyses are based on their statistical notes. Wherever possible sex comparisons are based on age-adjusted rates of utilization. In comparing different types of facilities, we have tried to use similar utilization indices. But mental health facilities often use different procedures to measure and

ISBN 0-12-310850-0

report utilization, with a variety of indices, such as admissions, additions, discharges, and patient-care episodes. Definitions of the indices can be found in the appendix at the end of this chapter.

TYPES OF MENTAL HEALTH FACILITIES IN STUDY

State and County Mental Hospitals

Of the general treatment facilities to be discussed, state and county mental hospitals[1] have existed for the longest time. These hospitals were the primary resource, and in some cases the only resource, for the care and treatment of the mentally ill up through the 1940s.[1] The number of other facilities, such as outpatient clinics or general hospital inpatient psychiatric units, was very small. State and county mental hospitals had a large number of long-term, chronically ill patients.

Since 1950, there has been a decline in the use of state and county mental hospitals, both in absolute terms and as compared to other mental health facilities. This decline is due to innovations in treatment and rehabilitation of the mentally ill and to the opening and expansion of new types of facilities. As drugs and other therapies have been used to treat disorders such as schizophrenia, some patients who would previously have remained hospitalized are now able to return to the community. The growth of general hospital inpatient psychiatric units and community mental health centers has increased the number of facilities available for the mentally ill. The development of outpatient psychiatric units and halfway houses has made available alternate ways to treat those who do not need full hospitalization and also has aided in reintegrating patients into the community.

Despite this decline in the use of state and county mental hospitals, however, they still housed well over half of all psychiatric beds in the country in 1974. And because they have predominated for so long and generally have more complete records than other types of facilities, state and county mental hospitals have traditionally provided the basis for studies of mental health problems.

[1] This description is based on information contained in the following publications: Pollack, E. S., & Taube, C. A. Trends and projections in state hospital use, In J. Zusman & E. F. Bertsch (Eds.), *The future role of the state hospital.* Lexington, Mass.: D. C. Heath, 1975; Kramer, M., Taube, C. A., & Redick, R. Patterns of use of psychiatric facilities by the aged: Past, present, and future. In Eisdorfer, C. & Lawton, M. P. (Eds.), *The psychology of adult development and aging.* Washington, D.C.: American Psychological Association, 1973.

Community Mental Health Centers

Community mental health centers,[2] financed through federal funding provided under the Community Mental Health Centers Construction Act passed in 1963, were established as part of a governmental effort to make mental health services more readily available to the general population. They were designed to provide comprehensive mental health care while allowing the patient to remain close to home and retain his ties with his family and the community. Community mental health centers are set up on a catchment area basis. Each center serves a defined population group no smaller than 75,000 nor larger than 200,000 people.

Because community mental health centers operate on the local level, their services vary depending on the needs of the community. However, in order to qualify for federal funding, all community mental health centers must provide inpatient care, outpatient care, 24-hour-a-day emergency service, and consultation and education services for community agencies and professional personnel. Additional functions often performed include diagnostic services, rehabilitation, precare and aftercare, and research and evaluation. The community mental health center may furnish special services to particular groups in the area such as children, the elderly, or alcoholics, or implement programs to combat specific local problems such as child abuse, suicide, or juvenile delinquency.

Outpatient psychiatric services[3] are made available through clinics and generally are directed to patients who do not require hospitalization. These clinics provide a variety of services, including aftercare treatment for those who were previously hospitalized, so as to prevent their rehospitalization and help them achieve a maximum level of functioning; diagnostic services to determine a person's needs and proper placement; special education services for children unable to participate in the regular school system; and vocational rehabilitation. In addition, such clinics usually fulfill research, education, and training activities by acting as consultants to community agencies, offering general public education and in-service training for both their own staff and the staff of community agencies, and making program evaluations.

[2] The information for this description was taken from the following publications: Kramer, M., Rosen, B. M., & Willis, E. M. Definitions and distributions of mental disorders in a racist society. In *Racism and mental health.* In Willie, C. V., Kramer, B. M., & Brown, B. S. (Eds) University of Pittsburgh Press, Pittsburgh: 1973; Kramer, M., Taube, C. A., & Redick, R. W. Patterns of use of psychiatric facilities by the aged: Past, present, and future. In Eisdorfer, C., & Lawton, M. (Eds.), *The psychology of adult development and aging.* Washington, D.C.: *American Psychological Association,* 1973.

[3] This description is based on information contained in: National Institute of Mental Health. *Outpatient psychiatric services, 1971–72.* Washington, D.C.: U.S. Government Printing Office, 1973.

General Hospital Inpatient Psychiatric Units

General hospital inpatient psychiatric units[4] provide mental health services within general hospitals that serve patients requiring short-term hospitalization. These units may be operated as separate inpatient services, in which there are a number of beds reserved exclusively for psychiatric patients, who are kept separate from the other patients in the hospital; or as general inpatient services, in which the psychiatric, medical, and surgical patients share the same facilities. In most cases our data deal only with the separate inpatient services.

The number of psychiatric services in general hospitals has grown rapidly since World War II. Whereas in 1939 only 37 general hospitals and 6 Veterans Administration hospitals had psychiatric inpatient services, 766 general hospitals had separate inpatient psychiatric facilities by 1970. Why this major expansion? Some of it may be attributed to the increased coverage of mental illness costs by health insurance, Medicare, and Medicaid; and the earmarking of funds for the construction of psychiatric beds. In addition, the passage of the federal Community Mental Health Centers Construction Act in 1963 encouraged the creation of general hospital psychiatric units, since about half of the inpatient services for community mental health centers are provided by general hospitals.

General hospital inpatient psychiatric units are operated by the Veterans Administration, state or local governments, or nongovernmental groups. Veterans hospitals generally have the largest psychiatric wards. Although they account for only 12% of the psychiatric inpatient units, the veterans hospitals house over one-third of the psychiatric beds.

Private Mental Hospitals

Private mental hospitals[5] are mental health facilities run by nongovernmental agencies or administrations, either as profit-making or nonprofit institutions. As a rule, nonprofit private mental hospitals are run

[4] This description is based on information contained in the following publications: National Institute of Mental Health. *Psychiatric services in general hospitals, 1969–1970* (DHEW Publication No. HSM 72-139). Washington, D.C.: U.S. Government Printing Office 1972; Taube, C. A. *Increases in general hospital psychiatric inpatient services.* Washington, D.C.: U.S. Government Printing Office 1969; Bachrach, L. L. *Marital status of discharges from psychiatric units of general hospitals, United States, 1970–71: I. analysis by age, color, and sex* (DHEW Publication No. HSM 73-9005). Washington, D.C.: U.S. Government Printing Office 1973.

[5] This description is based on information contained in: National Institute of Mental Health. *Private mental hospitals, 1969–70* (DHEW Publication No. HSM 72-9809). Washington, D.C.: U.S. Government Printing Office, 1972.

by churches or other nonprofit organizations, whereas individuals, partnerships, or corporations generally operate profit-making hospitals.

In January 1970, there were 149 private mental hospitals reporting data to the National Institute of Mental Health. Although the greater number of these hospitals were run for profit—over one-half—the nonprofit private mental hospitals were larger. Many private mental hospitals have restrictions as to the types of patients they will admit. Nearly half of the hospitals have diagnostic restrictions, with mentally retarded patients the most often excluded. Over 60% of the private mental hospitals have age restrictions, setting a minimum age requirement ranging anywhere from 11 to 14.

Children's Mental Health Facilities

Children's mental health facilities[6] may be those designed exclusively for children, or they may serve children within an institution also used for adults. Although all psychiatric facilities previously discussed (except for the psychiatric wards of veterans hospitals) treat children, our analysis of children's facilities is restricted to data from state and county mental hospitals, general hospital inpatient psychiatric units, outpatient psychiatric units and facilities that serve children exclusively. The final category includes hospital inpatient treatment units for emotionally disturbed children and psychiatric hospitals for children. Children admitted to a facility that also treats adults may be placed on wards with patients of all ages or sent to live in separate units.

The hospital inpatient treatment units discussed in our data on children's mental health facilities are small psychiatric facilities within private, state, and county mental hospitals. Residential treatment centers designed exclusively for children generally treat those who are mildly to moderately disturbed, whereas psychiatric hospitals for children, more psychiatrically and medically oriented than the residential treatment centers, usually treat children manifesting more serious types of disturbances.

[6] The information for this description is taken from the following publications: National Institute of Mental Health. *Residential psychiatric facilities for children and adolescents, United States, 1971–72* (DHEW Publication No. ADM 74-78). Washington, D.C.: U.S. Government Printing Office 1972; National Institute of Mental Health. *Hospital inpatient treatment units for emotionally disturbed children, United States, 1971–72* (DHEW Publication No. ADM 74-82). Washington, D.C.: U.S. Government Printing Office 1972; Redick, R. W. *Utilization of psychiatric facilities by persons uner 18 years of age, United States, 1971.* (DHEW Publication No. NIH 74-655). Washington, D.C.: U.S. Government Printing Office 1973.

DEMOGRAPHIC CHARACTERISTICS OF PATIENT POPULATIONS

Men and women entered mental health facilities at virtually equal rates overall during the years studied. Had we restricted our examination to certain kinds of facilities, however, the entry rates for men and women would not have been so similar. For instance, men utilized state and county mental hospitals, the facilities most commonly studied, at a higher rate than did women. Men were also overrepresented at inpatient units in general hospitals. However, women's rate of use of private mental hospitals was higher than men's, while the sexes were about equally represented at community mental health centers and outpatient psychiatric services. Table 1.1 shows the rates at which males and females utilized five types of general treatment facilities during a period in the early 1970s.

Utilization of mental health facilities was generally low among adolescents and the elderly, with the highest utilization rates found among those in middle adulthood. This can be seen in Figures 1.1–1.5, in which utilization rates are plotted against age at each of the five types of general treatment facilities. For state and county mental hospitals, community mental health centers, outpatient psychiatric services and general hospital inpatient psychiatric units, rates are shown separately for white males, white females, nonwhite males, and nonwhite females; at private mental hospitals there is no breakdown by color.

Table 1.2 shows the utilization rates of white males, white females, nonwhite males, and nonwhite females at each of the five types of general treatment facilities. Within three groups of facilities (state and county mental hospitals, community mental health centers, and outpatient psychiatric services), nonwhites of each sex had a higher utilization rate than did whites of the same sex. On the other hand, whites, regardless of sex, had the higher rates at private mental hospitals. At general hospital inpatient psychiatric units, the utilization rates of nonwhite males exceeded that of white males, while the white females rate surpassed that of nonwhite females. Referring once more to Figures 1.1 through 1.5, it can be seen that the utilization rate of nonwhite males in state and county mental hospitals and general hospital inpatient psychiatric units far outstrips that of white males and females and of nonwhite females, particularly during the peak utilization years of middle adulthood. At community mental health centers, the difference in utilization rates is more striking as to the race variable than the sex variable. With outpatient psychiatric services, both race and sex differences in utilization rates are quite noticeable. The utilization of most mental health facilities showed a relationship between low income level and utilization rate. Men and women with the highest utiliza-

TABLE 1.1

Admission Rates of Males and Females at General Treatment Facilities

AGE-ADJUSTED RATES OF ADMISSIONS[a] PER 100,000 POPULATION	STATE AND COUNTY MENTAL HOSPITALS		COMMUNITY MENTAL HEALTH CENTERS		OUTPATIENT PSYCHIATRIC SERVICES		GENERAL HOSPITAL INPATIENT PSYCHIATRIC UNITS		PRIVATE MENTAL HOSPITALS	
	MALE	FEMALE	MALE	FEMALE	MALE	FEMALE	MALE	FEMALE	MALE	FEMALE
	253.4	143.3	1058.4	1078.8	635.8	649.0	320.1	261.8	34.6	47.1
Year	1972		1973		1971		1970–71		1970	

[a]At community mental health centers, addition rates are used. At general hospital inpatient psychiatric units, discharge rates are used.

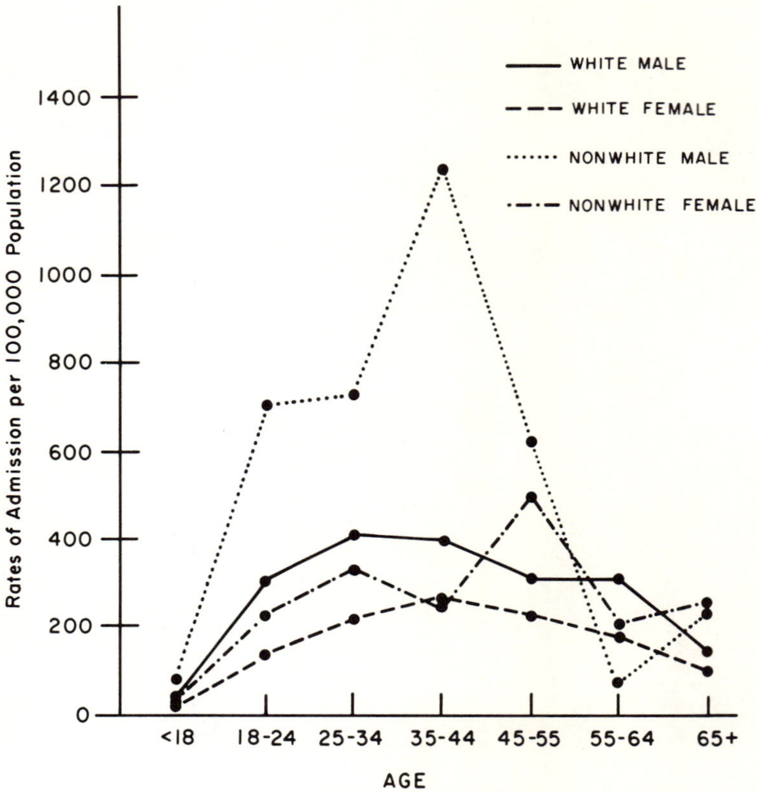

FIGURE 1.1. Admission rates at state and county mental hospitals in 1972, broken down by sex, color, and age. (Sources for this and the following figures can be found at the end of Chapter 1.)

tion rates at state and county mental hospitals and outpatient psychiatric services were in the lowest income group (not shown).

Marital status was also found to be highly correlated with rates of utilization at the four types of facilities for which these data were available. Separated or divorced men and women used each type of mental health facility more frequently than did men and women in other marital statuses. This can be seen in Figure 1.6, which presents utilization rates broken down by sex and marital status. (Note that the scale of rates is different for three of the four types of facilities shown.) For all facilities, men who were separated, divorced, or widowed had higher rates of utilization than did women who were separated, divorced, or widowed. Except in state and county mental hospitals, married women had higher rates of treatment than did married men. Among men in each type of facility, those who were separated or divorced had the highest rate of utilization; married men the

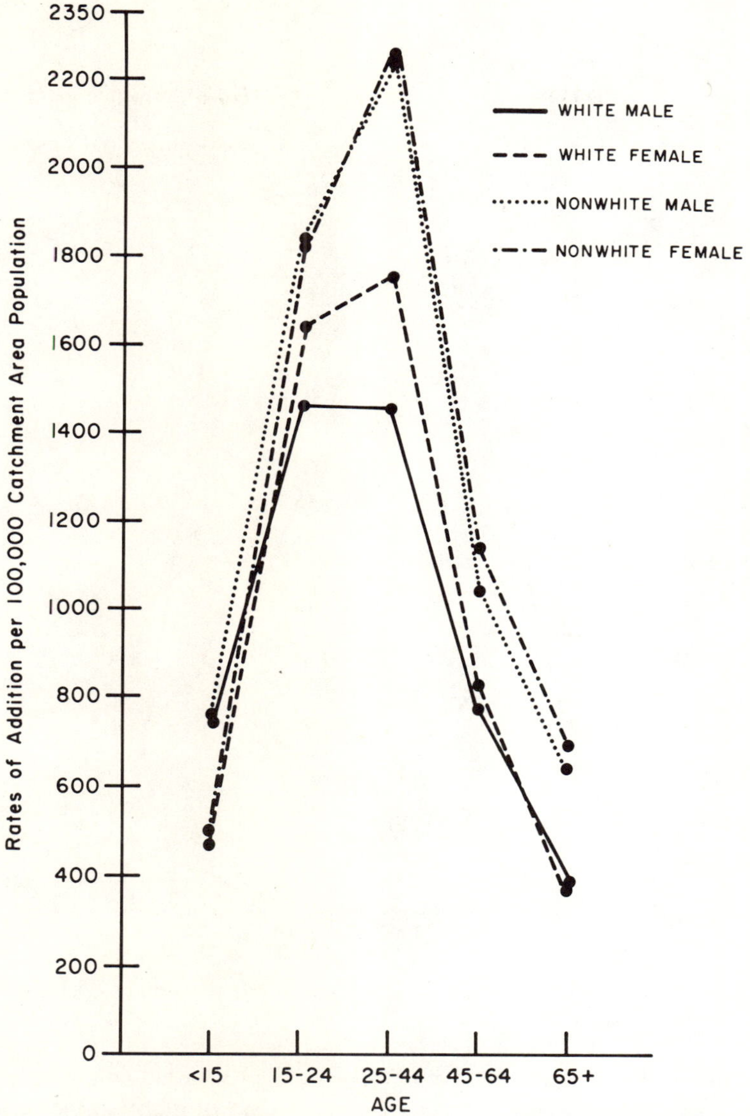

FIGURE 1.2. Addition rates at community mental health centers in 1973, broken down by sex, color, and age.

lowest; with the widowed and never-married men falling in between the two extremes. Among women, those separated or divorced had the highest rate of utilization in each type of facility, but the other three marital statuses showed no consistent rate magnitude from facility to facility.

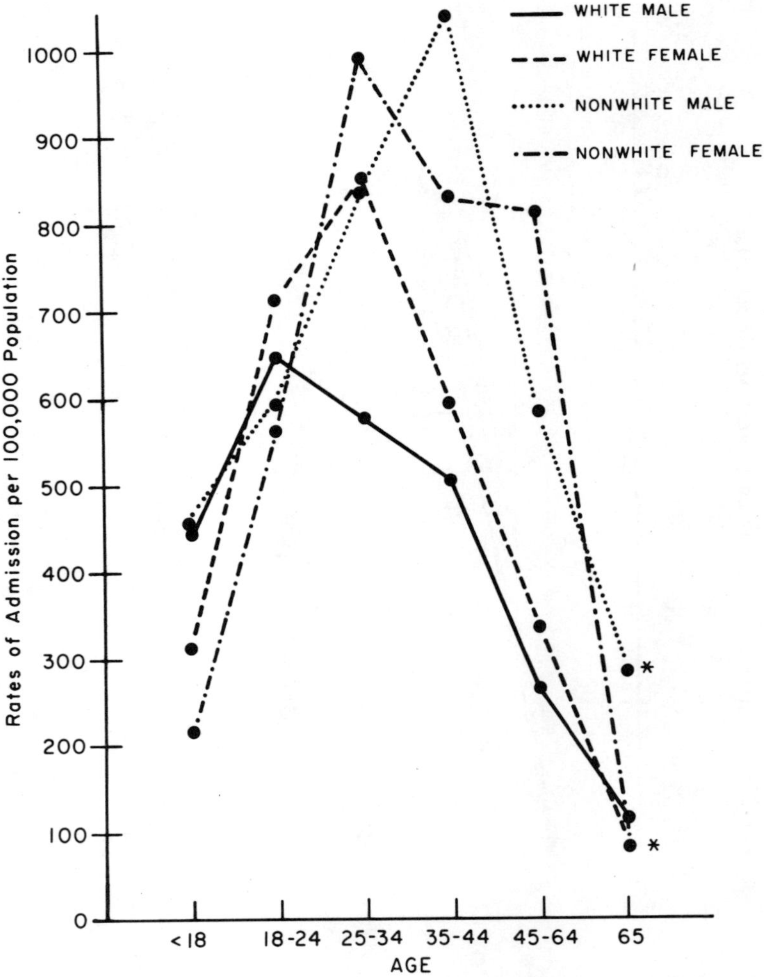

FIGURE 1.3. Admission rates at outpatient psychiatric services in 1969, broken down by sex, color, and age.

One of the most alarming findings of this project was the high rate of mental health facilities utilization by women who headed families without spouses. For instance, Figure 1.7 shows that in 1970 women who headed families were admitted to outpatient psychiatric services at a rate which exceeded one admission for every 100 female family heads in the population. The admission rate of divorced and single female family heads was similarly high (not shown). Women who were separated from their husbands and headed families had an admission rate of over 3 per 100 of the population. Widowed female family heads, however, appeared far less vulner-

TABLE 1.2
Utilization Rates by Sex and Color

	WHITE MALES	NONWHITE MALES	WHITE FEMALES	NONWHITE FEMALES
State and County Mental Hospitals (Admissions, 1972)	228.5	425.2	136.5	190.1
Community Mental Health Centers (Additions, 1973)	1014.9	1326.3	1049.9	1256.7
Outpatient Psychiatric Services (Admissions, 1969)	417.6	587.9	434.8	503.5
General Hospital Inpatient Psychiatric Units (Discharges, 1970–1971)	297.0	481.8	265.5	236.2
Private Mental Hospitals (Admissions, 1971)	39.1	14.1	53.5	16.1

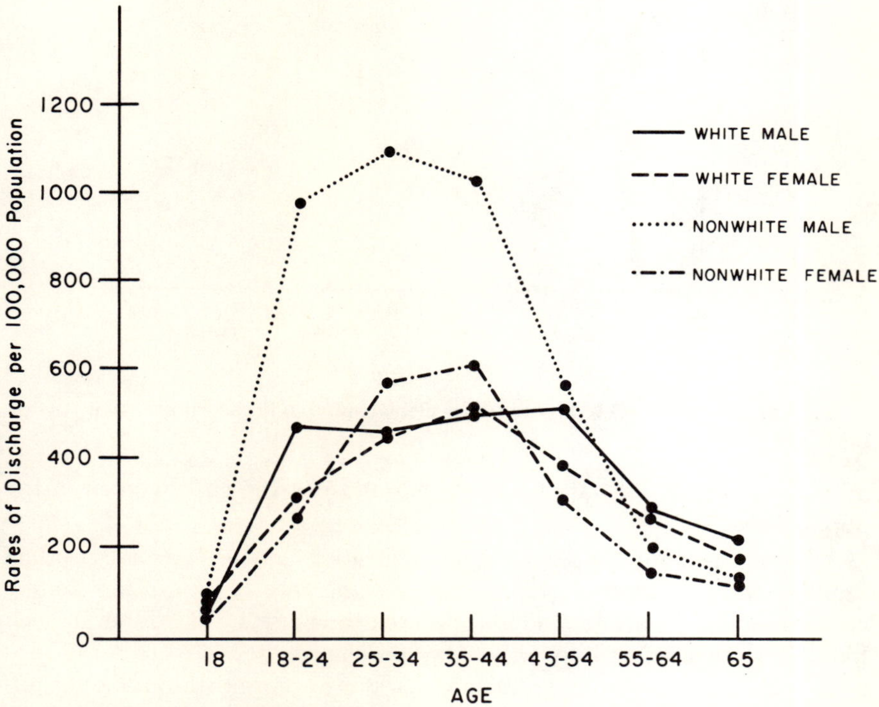

FIGURE 1.4 Discharge rates at general hospital inpatient psychiatric units in 1970–1971, broken down by sex, color, and age.

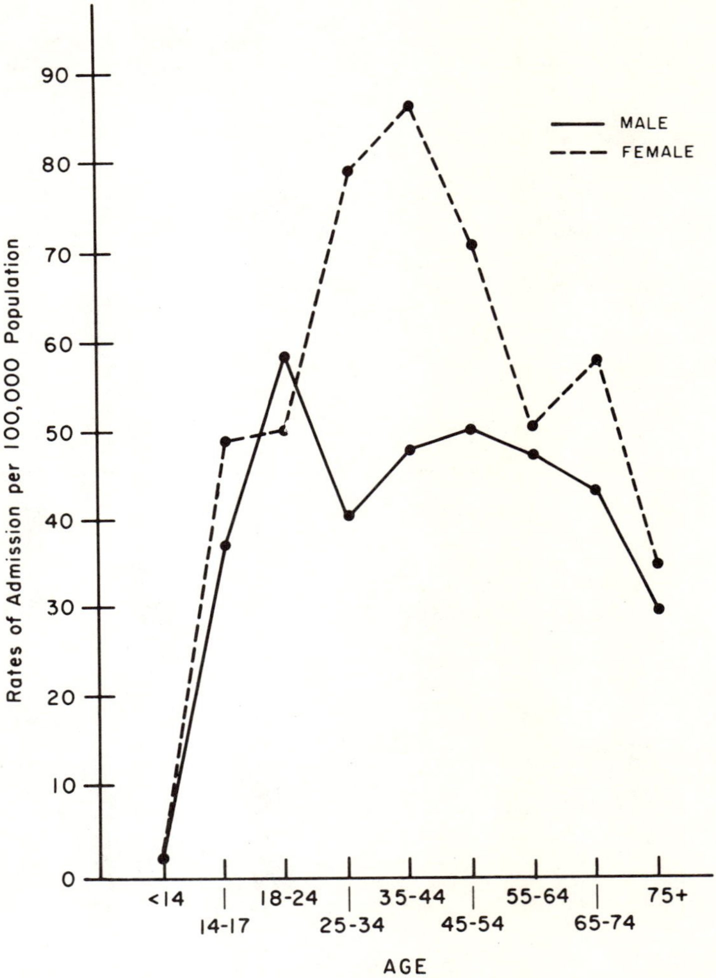

FIGURE 1.5. Admission rates at private mental hospitals in 1970, broken down by sex and age.

able. Their utilization rate was less than 0.3 per 100 such women in the population.

These startlingly high rates of utilization among women heading families without spouses were echoed in the rate of utilization among children in female-headed families, as seen in Figure 1.7. Children in such families were admitted to outpatient psychiatric services at a rate approaching one admission per 100 population, or more than double the admission rate of children in husband–wife families. At state and county mental hospitals, as indicated in Figure 1.8, admission rates of women who

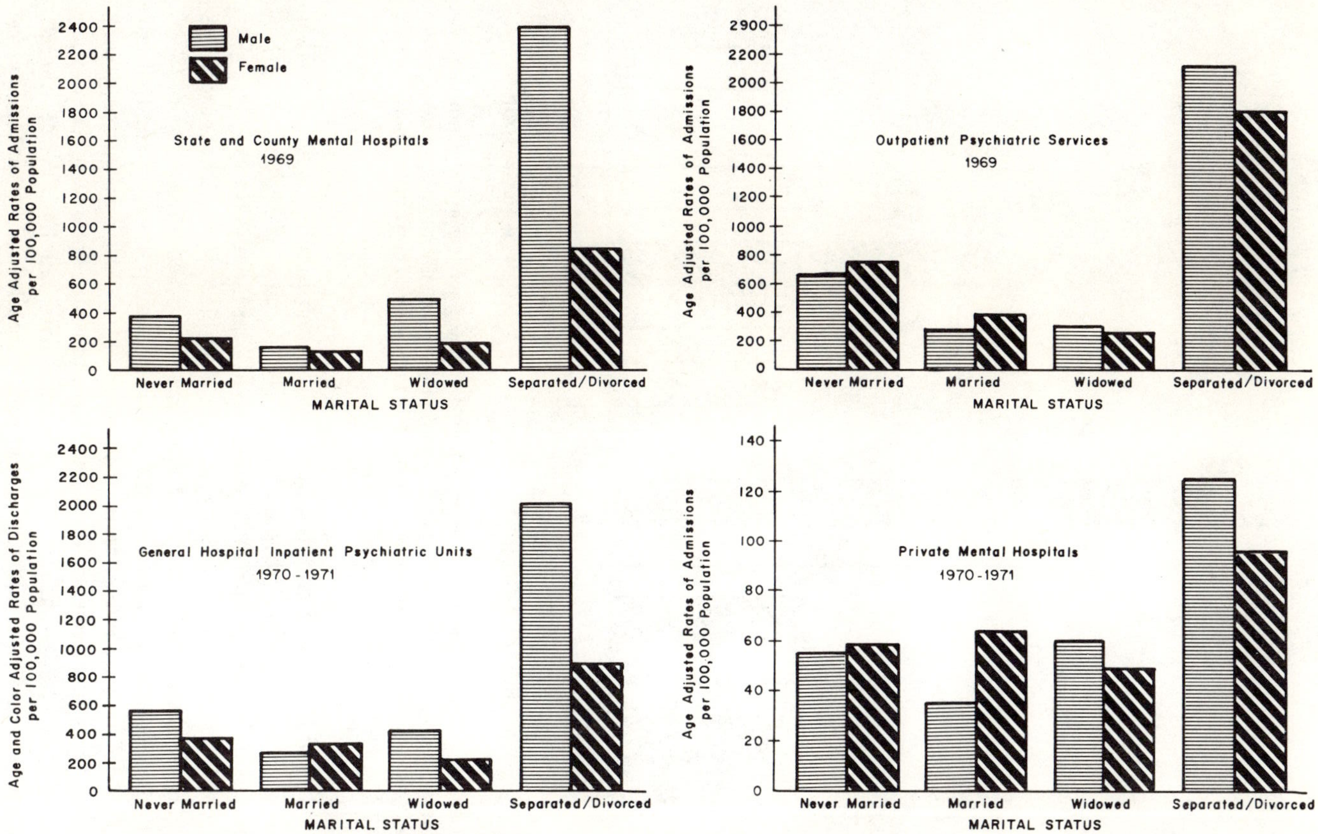

FIGURE 1.6. Utilization rates at four types of mental health facilities, broken down by sex and marital status.

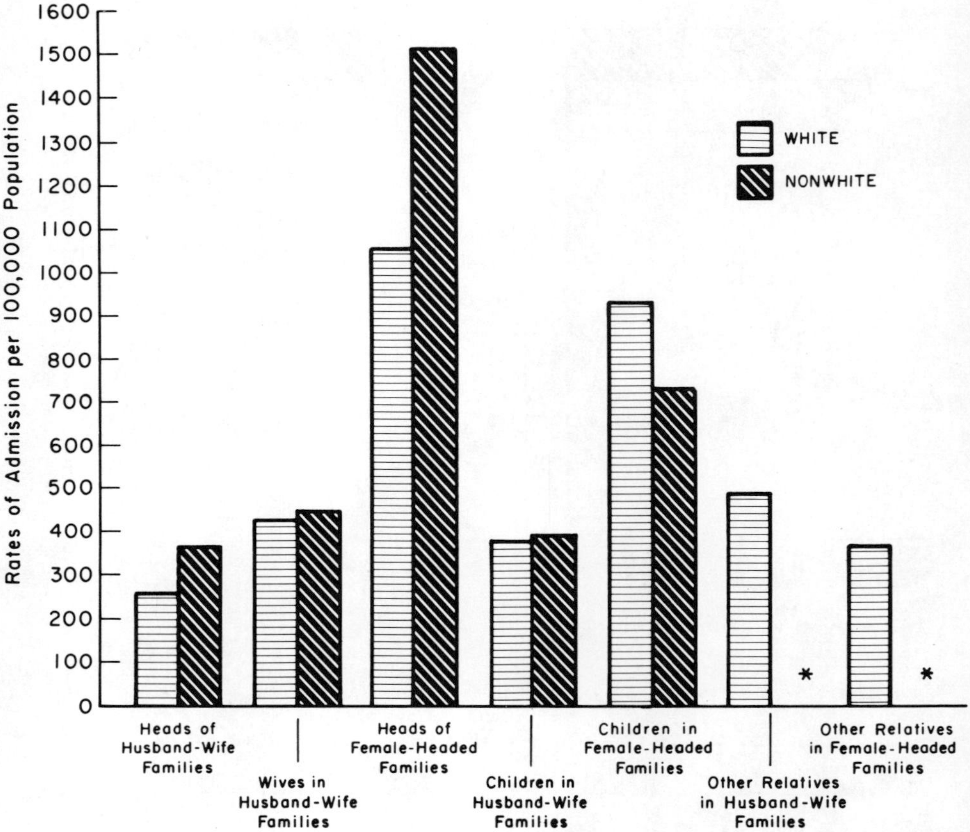

FIGURE 1.7. Admission rates at outpatient psychiatric services in 1970, broken down by type of family and relationship to family head. (Asterisks signify numbers were below accepted limits of reliability. Heads of husband-wife families are always male. Definitions of all family status terms are given in the appendix.)

headed families and of children in female-headed families again exceeded those of parents and children in husband-wife families, although "other relatives" in husband-wife families also had high admission rates.

The youngest children of single parent families appear to demonstrate the most significant effects. As Figure 1.9 shows, children aged 6–17 in female-headed families had an admission rate at outpatient psychiatric services more than double that of 6–17-year-old children in husband-wife families, while children under 6 had an admission rate which was four times that of children under 6 in husband-wife families. While overall utilization rates for children at various mental health facilities were positively correlated with the age of the child, peaking in middle or late

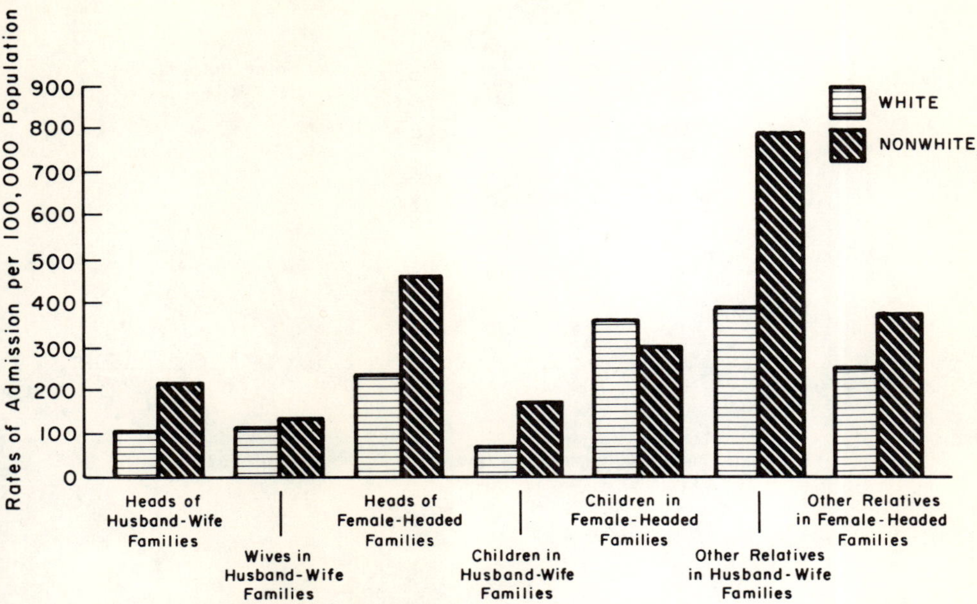

FIGURE 1.8. Admission rates at state and county mental hospitals in 1970, broken down by type of family and relationship to family head. (Heads of husband–wife families are always male. Definitions of all family status terms are given in the appendix.)

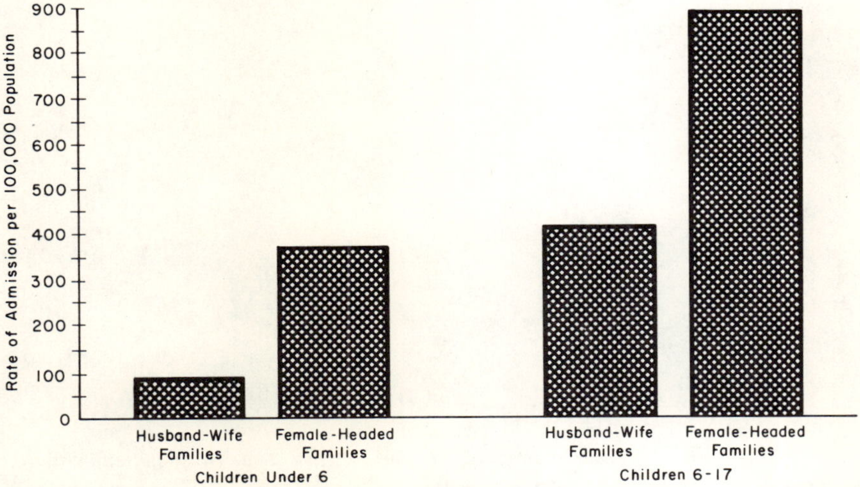

FIGURE 1.9. Admission rates of children at outpatient psychiatric services in 1970, broken down by type of family and age of child.

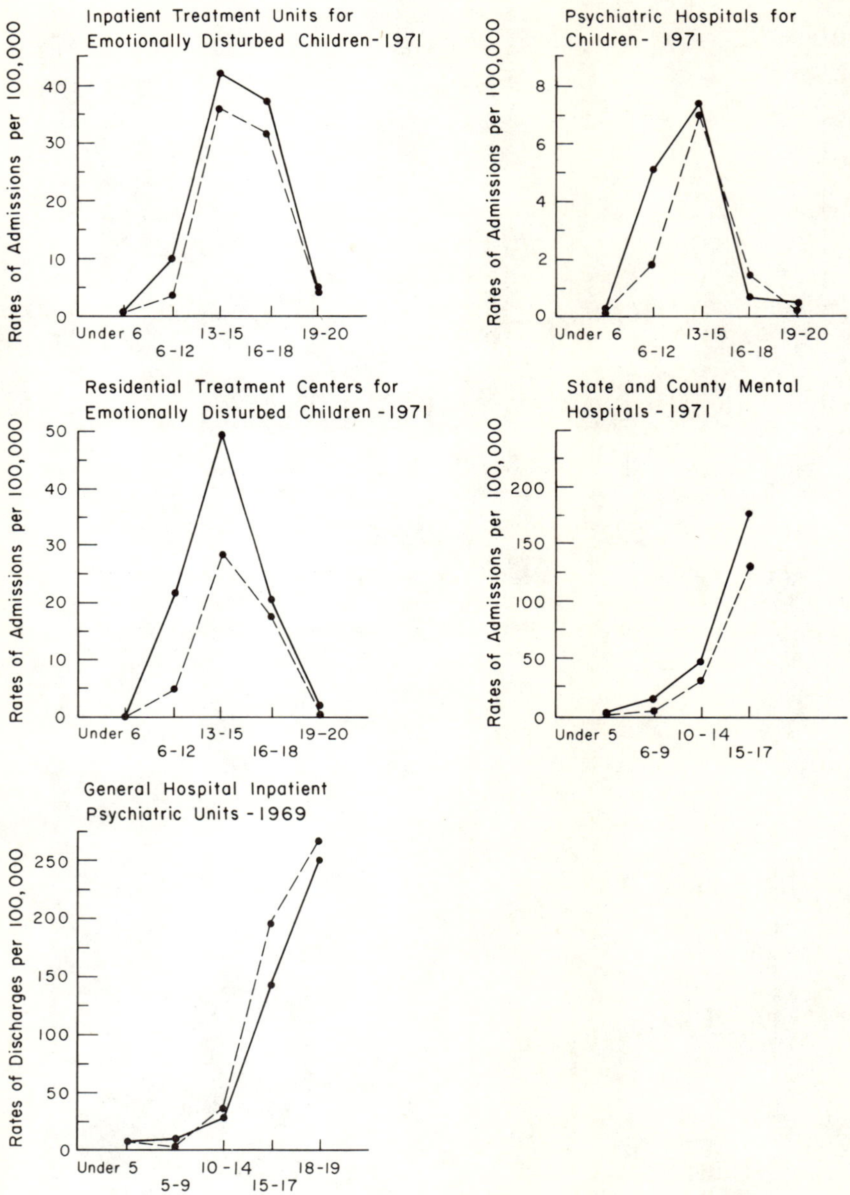

FIGURE 1.10. Utilization rates of children at five types of inpatient children's facilities, broken down by sex and age (Male ——, Female ---).

adolescence, children under 6 living with single-parent mothers who were separated, but not divorced from husbands, had a higher admission rate to outpatient psychiatric services than did children 6–13 living with such mothers. This reversal of the usual positive association of age and utilization rate should be a cause for concern.

In all children's facilities except for general hospital inpatient psychiatric units, male children had higher rates of utilization than did female children. In most instances these sex differences appear at every age level, as can be seen in Figure 1.10. Two predominant patterns of utilization by age appear. At inpatient treatment units, psychiatric hospitals for children, and residential treatment centers, utilization rates increase from ages under 6 to ages 13–15 and decline thereafter. In the two other types of facilities, utilization rates generally increase monotonically with age.

SUMMARY

This comparison of utilization rates across subgroups of the population based on data from the National Institute of Mental Health points to those groups most likely to be treated for mental illness. In general, men and women in middle adulthood, particularly those in low-income categories and those who are separated or divorced, are high utilization groups. Women heading families without spouses have a particularly high rate of treatment for mental illness. Sex differences vary across facilities, but nonwhite males have higher rates than do nonwhite females or whites of either sex in all facilities except private mental hospitals.

Although this analysis of utilization rates allows us to compare *treatment* rates among populations, it does not allow us to compare actual rates of mental illness. Those groups with the highest rates of treatment at mental health facilities do *not* necessarily have the highest rates of mental illness, since rates of utilization reflect selection processes for treatment among and within communities, as well the extent of mental illness in the communities.

APPENDIX

Definitions of Indices of Utilization[7]

Utilization indices described here reflect the incidence of movement into and out of mental health facilities. The indices defined here are used in Chapters 1 and 2.

[7] These definitions were adapted from a variety of National Institute of Mental Health publications including Bachrach, L. *General characteristics of additions to federally funded community mental health centers during 1971,* (DHEW Publication No. NIH 74–655). Washington, D.C.: U.S. Government Printing

Admissions

Admissions include both first admissions and readmissions as well as returns from short-term leaves and transfers from non-inpatient facilities. Returns from extended leaves such as convalescent leaves, conditional discharges, and family care are not counted as admissions. Admissions is a duplicated count, meaning that a person is counted as an admission each time he enters a facility.

Additions

As defined by all facilities other than community mental health centers, additions include admissions and returns from extended leave. Community mental health centers define additions as an unduplicated count. Thus a patient admitted more than once during the period studied is counted as a single addition.

Discharges

A discharge occurs when a patient is removed from the hospital books. They include transfers and extended leaves. In some studies, deaths are included; and in others they are not. In all cases, a discharge is a duplicated count. If a person is discharged more than once, each discharge is counted separately.

Terminations

Terminations appear to be used primarily by outpatient facilities as opposed to discharges, used by inpatient facilities. A person has terminated his care if he has discontinued services at his own volition or if he has not been seen for 90 days.

Definitions of Family Statuses[8]

The following terms are used in Figures 1.7 and 1.8 of Chapter 1.

Household means all related and/or unrelated persons who occupy a house, apartment, group of rooms, or a single room occupied as separate living quarters.

Family is two or more persons living in the same household who are related by blood, marriage, or adoption.

Head of Family is the person in the family who is regarded as head by the members of the family. Although this definition implies that the head of a husband–wife family could be the wife, a married woman is not classified as head if the husband is present.

Wives in husband–wife families include both legally married and common-law wives.

Children of family head include stepchildren and adopted children as well as biological children.

Other relative of family head means any person who is related to the family head by blood, marriage, or adoption other than the wife or child of the head.

Office, 1973; Witkin, M. *Outpatient psychiatric services 1971–1972,* (DHEW Publication No. ADM 74-69). Washington, D.C.: U.S. Government Printing Office, 1973; National Institute of Mental Health. *Socioeconomic characteristics of admissions to inpatient services of state and county mental hospitals, 1969* (DHEW Publications No. HSM 72-9048). Washington, D.C.: U.S. Government Printing Office, 1971.

[8] These definitions were adapted from Redick, R. W., & Johnson, C. *Marital status, living arrangements and family characteristics of admissions to state and county mental hospitals and outpatient psychiatric clinics, United States, 1970* (DHEW Publication No. ADM 74-6). Washington, D.C.: U.S. Government Printing Office, 1973.

SOURCES FOR FIGURES IN CHAPTER 1

Figure 1.1. (Numbers are from Table 8 in the National Institute of Mental Health publication, Taube, C. A., *Readmissions to inpatient services of State and County Mental Hospitals,* 1972. Washington, D.C.: U.S. Government Printing Office [For the purposes of this graph, only the numbers in the "all admissions" columns were included. Rates were calculated from these numbers.])

Figure 1.2. (Most of these rates were reported in Table 1 of the National Institute of Mental Health publication, Redick, R. W. *Addition rates to federally funded community mental health centers, United States, 1973. Washington, D.C.: U.S. Government Printing Office* [Statistics in this table were used to calculate adjusted rates. Based on reports from 261 community mental health centers.])

Figure 1.3. (Numbers are reported in Table 1 of the National Institute of Mental Health publication, *Socio-economic characteristics of admissions to outpatient psychiatric services, 1969. Washington, D.C.: U.S. Government Printing Office* [Rates were calculated from statistics reported in this table.])

Figure 1.4. (Numbers are reported in Table 1 of the National Institute of Mental Health publication, Taube, C. A., *Differential utilization of general hospital psychiatric inpatient units by whites and nonwhites, United States, 1970–1971. Washington, D.C.: U.S. Government Printing Office* [Rates were calculated from these numbers. Although some rates are reported in the source, in order to maintain consistency, these rates were recalculated using the same resident civilian population statistics used in the calculation of adjusted rates. As the source indicates, "these data are derived from a sample survey of discharges during the month of February, 1971. Estimates shown . . . represent a year's discharges centering on this month (e.g. September 1970-August 1971)." 1971 population statistics were used in the calculation of rates.])

Figure 1.5. (Rates are based on numbers reported in Table 1 of the National Institute of Mental Health publication, Taube, C. A., *Admissions to private mental hospitals, 1970. Washington, D.C.: U.S. Government Printing Office* [All rates have been computed from the calculated numbers. According to the source, these numbers are "based on reports from 141 of the 160 private mental hospitals in operation as of November 1970."])

Figure 1.6. (Numbers and most rates for state and county mental hospitals are reported in Tables C and D of the National Institute of Mental Health publication, Taube, C. A., *Admission rates by age, sex and marital status, state and county mental hospitals, 1969. Washington, D.C.: U.S. Government Printing Office* [Adjusted rates were calculated from statistics, including population statistics, reported in these tables.] Numbers and some rates for general hospital inpatient psychiatric units are reported in Tables 2 and 3 respectively of the National Institute of Mental Health publication, Bachrach, L. L., *Marital status of discharges from psychiatric inpatient units of general hospitals, United States, 1970–1971: I. analysis by age, color and sex. Washington, D.C.: U.S. Government Printing Office* [Adjusted rates were calculated from these numbers. The population statistics reported in Table 1 of the source, and used in the calculation of the specific rates reported therein, were used to compute adjusted rates.] Numbers and rates for outpatient psychiatric services are reported in Table 7 of the National Institute of Mental Health publication, *Socio-economic characteristics of admissions to outpatient psychiatric services, 1969. Washington, D.C.: U.S. Government Printing Office* [Adjusted rates were calculated from these statistics using the same census statistics reported in the source to calculate the rates reported therein.] Rates for private mental hospitals are based on numbers reported in Table 2 of the National Institute of Mental Health publication, Taube, C. A., *Admissions to private mental hospitals,* 1970. *Washington, D.C.: U.S. Government Printing Office* [All rates have been computed from the calculated numbers. According to the source, these numbers are "based on reports from 141 of the 160 private mental hospitals in operations as of November 1970."])

Figure 1.7. (These rates are reported in Table 5 of the National Institute of Mental Health publication, Redick, R. W. & Johnson, C., *Marital status, living arrangements and family characteristics of admissions to state and county mental hospitals and outpatient psychiatric clinics, United States, 1970. Washington, D.C.: U.S. Government Printing Office* [Because most of these data either are not broken down by sex or are categorized so as to apply only to one sex, no adjusted rates were calculated.])

Figure 1.8. (These rates were reported in Table 4 of the National Institute of Mental Health publication, Redick, R. W. & Johnson, C., *Marital status, living arrangements and family characteristics of admissions to state and county mental hospitals and outpatient psychiatric clinics, United States 1970. Washington, D.C.: U.S. Government Printing Office* [Because most of these data either are not broken down by sex or are categorized so as to apply only to one sex, no adjusted rates were calculated.])

Figure 1.9. (These statistics are reported in Table 1 of the National Institute of Mental Health publication, Redick, R. W. & Johnson, C., *Marital status, living arrangements and family characteristics of admissions to state and county mental hospitals and outpatient psychiatric clinics, United States, 1970. Washington, D.C.: U.S. Government Printing Office.*

Figure 1.10. (Rates for inpatient treatment units were calculated from numbers reported in Table 8 of the National Institute of Mental Health publication, *Hospital inpatient treatment units for emotionally disturbed children, United States, 1971–1972. Washington, D.C.: U.S. Government Printing Office* [These statistics are, according to the source, based on 153 reporting units.] Rates for residential treatment centers are based on numbers reported in Table 7 of the National Institute of Mental Health publication, *Residential psychiatric facilities for children and adolescents, United States, 1971–1972. Washington, D.C.: U.S. Government Printing Office* Rates for general hospital inpatient psychiatric units are calculated from numbers reported in Table 18 of the National Institute of Mental Health publication, *Psychiatric services in general·hospitals, 1969–1970. Washington, D.C.: U.S. Government Printing Office* Rates for psychiatric hospitals for children were calculated from numbers reported in Table N of the National Institute of Mental Health publication, *Residential psychiatric facilities for children and adolescents, United States, 1971–1972. Washington, D.C.: U.S. Government Printing Office* Rates for state and county mental hospitals are based on numbers reported in Table 1 of the National Institute of Mental Health publication, Taube, C. A. & Meyer, N. G., *Children and state mental hospitals.*)

Chapter 2

PATTERNS OF DIAGNOSES RECEIVED BY MEN AND WOMEN

Deborah Belle
Noreen Goldman

Chapter 1 examined utilization rates at mental health facilities to discern which demographic groups appear to run the greatest risk of mental health problems—at least those mental health problems that do receive treatment. This chapter explores the specific diagnoses made when men and women were treated for mental health problems. Again, utilization rates will be examined, this time diagnosis-specific utilization rates. Four important diagnoses will receive particular attention: drug disorders, alcohol disorders, depressive disorders, and schizophrenia.

Among the different types of mental health facilities, there is considerable variation in the proportion of patients diagnosed as suffering from one of these four disorders. As Figure 2.1 shows, only about one-quarter of all patients at outpatient psychiatric services and less than one-half of all patients at community mental health centers were diagnosed with these conditions; yet at private mental hospitals, state and county mental hospitals, and general hospital inpatient psychiatric units, most patients were placed in one of these four diagnostic categories. Similar across-facility differences can be seen for particular disorders. For instance, depressive disorders was a major diagnosis at private mental hospitals, accounting for about one-quarter of all male patients and nearly one-half of all female patients, while the same condition accounted for a considerably smaller proportion of diagnoses of male and female patients at outpatient psychiatric services and at state and county mental hospitals.

Even with these gross disparities amongst the various types of facilities as to proportion of diagnoses made of one of the four disorders, all the

ISBN 0-12-310850-0

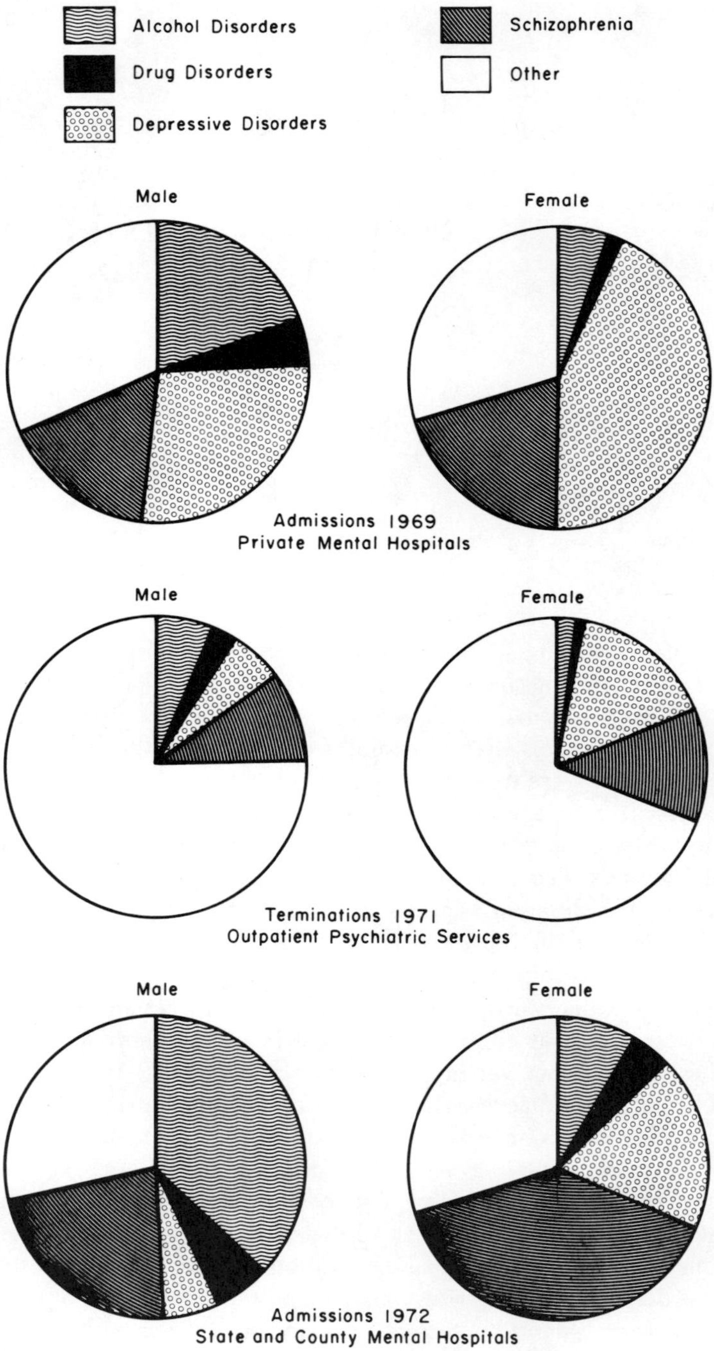

FIGURE 2.1. Distribution of patients by diagnosis at five major types of mental health facilities, broken down by sex.

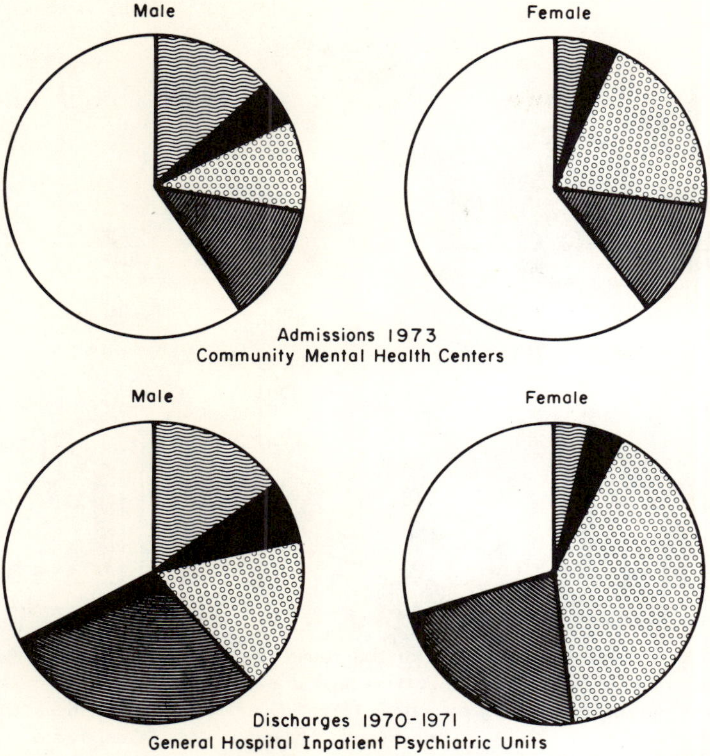

FIGURE 2.1—*Continued.* (*Depressive disorders* **is defined as "affective and depressive disorders" at state and county mental hospitals and as "psychotic depressive disorders and depressive neurosis" at general hospital inpatient psychiatric units. Sources for this and following figures can be found at the end of Chapter 2.)**

categories of facilities showed a clear pattern of sex differences in diagnoses. Figure 2.2 indicates that at each type of facility, the proportion of female patients diagnosed with depressive disorders was higher than the proportion of male patients diagnosed with depressive disorders, whereas the proportion of male patients diagnosed with alcohol or drug disorders was greater than the proportion of female patients so diagnosed. However, the proportion of male and female patients diagnosed with schizophrenia was remarkably similar at most types of facilities. The only exception was at state and county mental hospitals, where the proportion of female patients so diagnosed was noticeably higher than that of male patients. Because the information in Figure 2.1 reflects diagnoses of patients, the data do not reveal whether, within the general population, more males or females are likely to be treated for these mental disorders.

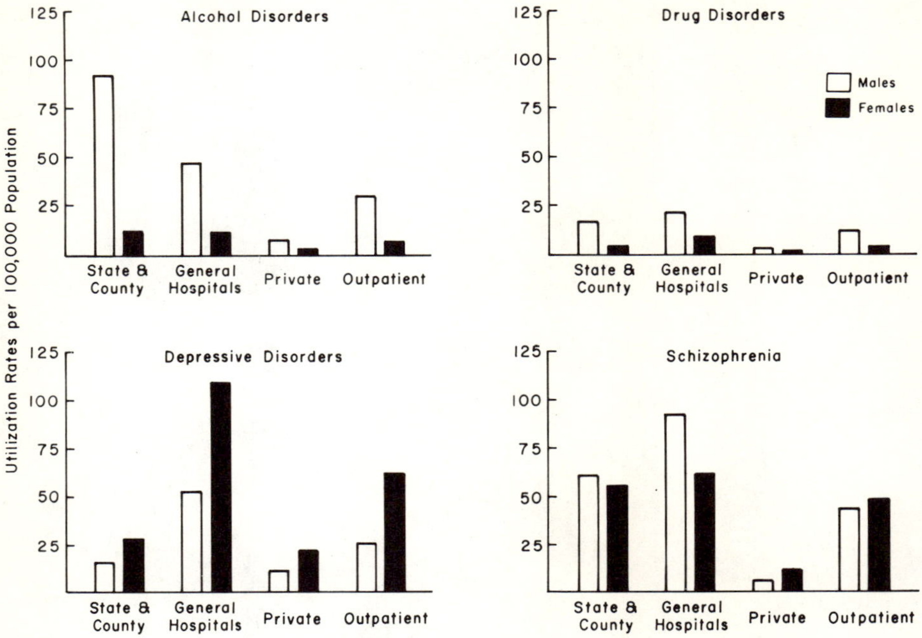

FIGURE 2.2. Utilization rates for four diagnoses at four types of mental health facilities, broken down by sex. (Utilization rates are as follows: state and county mental hospitals—age-adjusted admission rates, 1972; general hospital inpatient psychiatric units—discharge rates, 1970–1971; private mental hospitals—age-adjusted admissions rates, 1969; outpatient psychiatric services—age-adjusted terminations, 1971.)

Figure 2.2 shows utilization rates for those diagnosed with one of the four conditions at four major types of mental health facilities. These graphs show that among those with alcohol or drug problems, males had higher utilization rates than females at each of the four types of facilities, while in the depressive disorders category, females had higher utilization rates than males at each of the facilities. As to schizophrenia, male utilization rates exceeded female utilization rates at state and county mental hospitals and at general hospitals; the opposite was true at private hospitals and outpatient psychiatric services.

DRUG AND ALCOHOL DISORDERS

Figures 2.3 and 2.4 show age-specific rates of utilization for drug and alcohol disorders for the only types of facilities for which such information was available. With only a few exceptions, age-specific rates were considerably higher for males than for females for both diagnoses. Sex differences are particularly apparent at outpatient psychiatric services, where male utilization rates were approximately three times that of female utiliza-

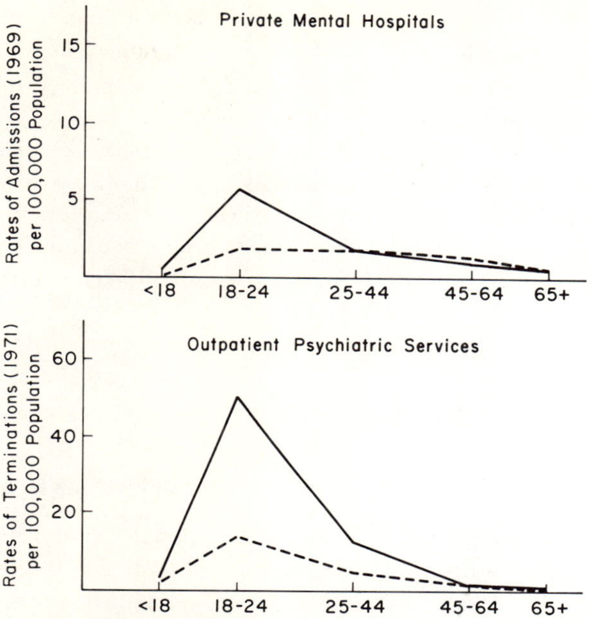

FIGURE 2.3. Utilization rates for drug disorders at two types of mental health facilities, broken down by age and sex (males —, females ---).

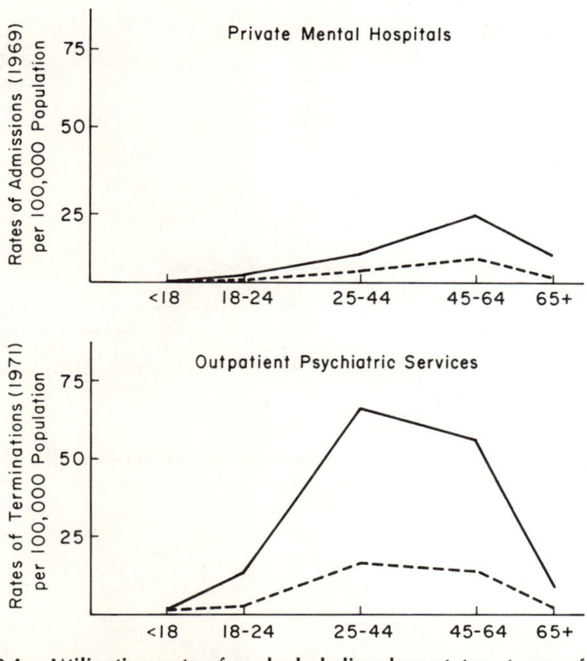

FIGURE 2.4. Utilization rates for alcohol disorders at two types of mental health facilities, broken down by age and sex (males —, females ---).

tion rates in the age group 18–24 for drug disorders, and in the age group 25–44 for alcohol disorders.

For males and females at both types of facilities, maximum utilization rates for drug disorders typically occurred in the 18–24 age group. In contrast, treatment for alcohol disorders reached its peak rate within an older group, with those aged 25–44 demonstrating the maximum utilization rate at outpatient psychiatric services and those aged 45–64 at private mental hospitals.

Whereas males show a large variation by age in utilization rates for both drug and alcohol disorders, female rates vary considerably less with age. A reverse pattern is seen for depressive disorders.

DEPRESSIVE DISORDERS

In each age group and type of facility females had higher rates of diagnosed depressive disorders than did males, with the sole exception of males aged 25–34 at state and county mental hospitals as shown in Figure 2.5. Sex differences were particularly marked at outpatient psychiatric services, with female rates for depressive disorders approximately triple those of males ages 25–44. Sex differences were least pronounced among the youngest ages and the oldest (under 18 and 65 and over).

While male utilization rates for depressive disorders did not vary greatly with age, female utilization rates for these disorders did show considerable variation with age. Females in the youngest and oldest groups had relatively low rates, reaching maximum rates in the age group 25–44 at both outpatient and private facilities, and at ages of 45–64 at state and county mental hospitals.

Sex differences were sharply pronounced within each subtype of depressive disorder: depressive neurosis, psychotic depressive disorders, and affective disorders. As shown in Figure 2.6, utilization rates of females exceeded those of males at the two types of facilities considered in almost all age groups for each of the three subtypes of depressive disorders. For both males and females, maximum utilization rates generally occur at

TABLE 2.1
Median Age of Male and Female Patients (By Subtype of Depressive Disorder)

SUBTYPE OF DEPRESSIVE DISORDER	STATE AND COUNTY MENTAL HOSPITALS (ADMISSIONS, 1972) MALE	FEMALE	OUTPATIENT PSYCHIATRIC SERVICES (TERMINATIONS, 1971) MALE	FEMALE
Depressive neurosis	36.8	36.6	33.6	34.0
Psychotic depressive disorders	41.7	43.3	43.1	42.0
Affective disorders	51.2	52.7	50.7	51.6

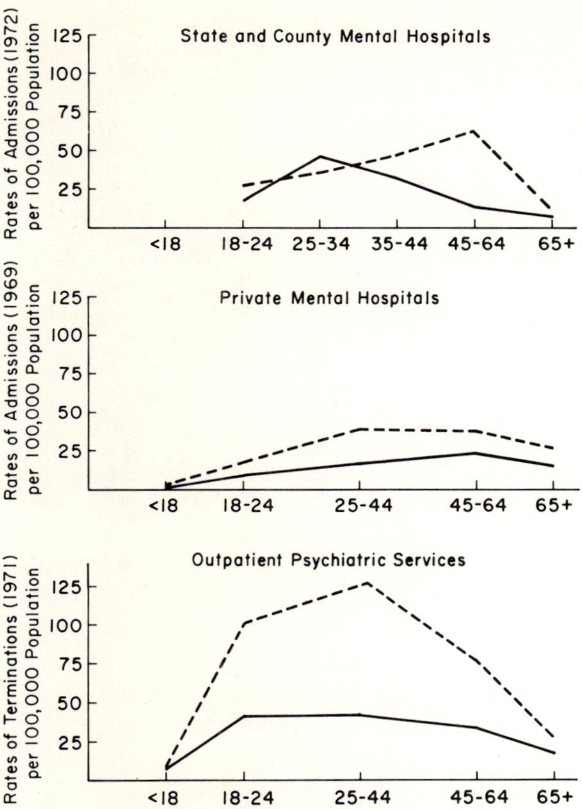

FIGURE 2.5. Utilization rates for depressive disorders at three types of mental health facilities, broken down by age and sex (males —, females---).

younger ages among those with depressive neurosis than those with either psychotic depressive disorders or affective disorders.

Data in Table 2.1 on median ages of those diagnosed as depressed show large age differences but practically no sex differences within subtypes of depression. Information from both state and county mental hospitals and outpatient psychiatric services (the only facilities for which such data were available) indicate that it is the younger patients who are diagnosed with depressive neurosis, while among older patients, whether male or female, there is a greater likelihood of diagnoses for the more severe types of depressive disorders.

SCHIZOPHRENIA

In contrast to the sharp sex differences which were found for drug disorders, alcohol disorders, and depressive disorders, sex differences in schizophrenia patients were minor. For the three types of facilities for

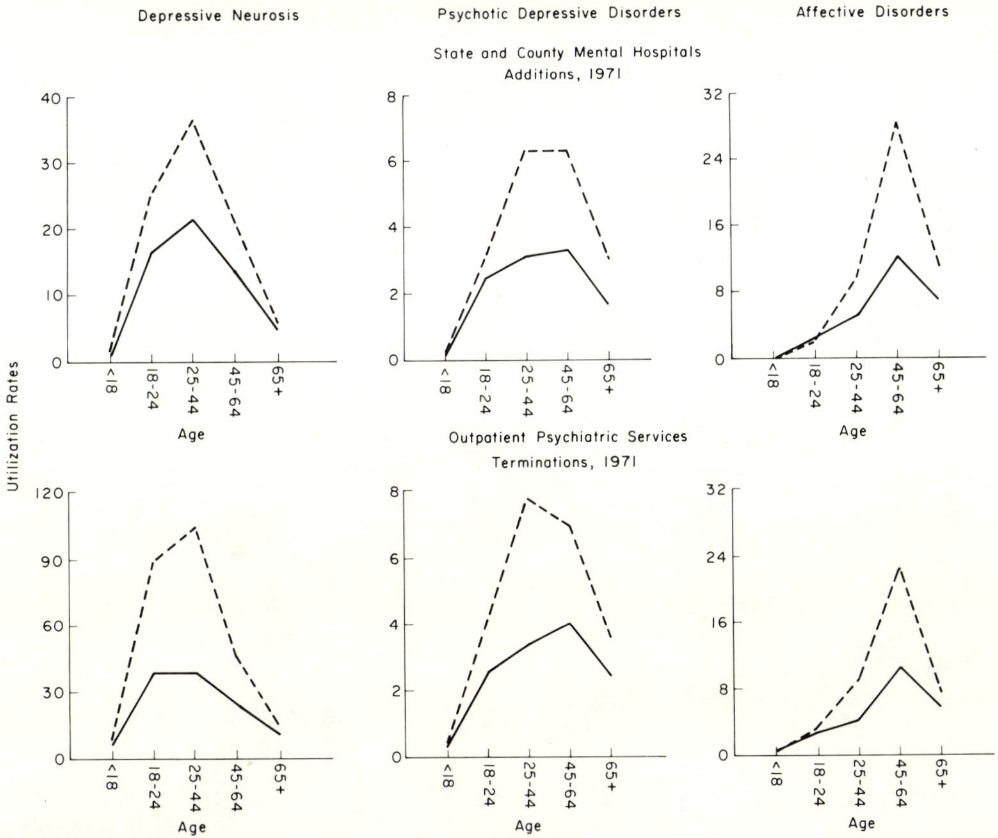

FIGURE 2.6. **Utilization rates for three subtypes of depressive disorders at two types of mental health facilities, broken down by age and sex (males—, females---).**

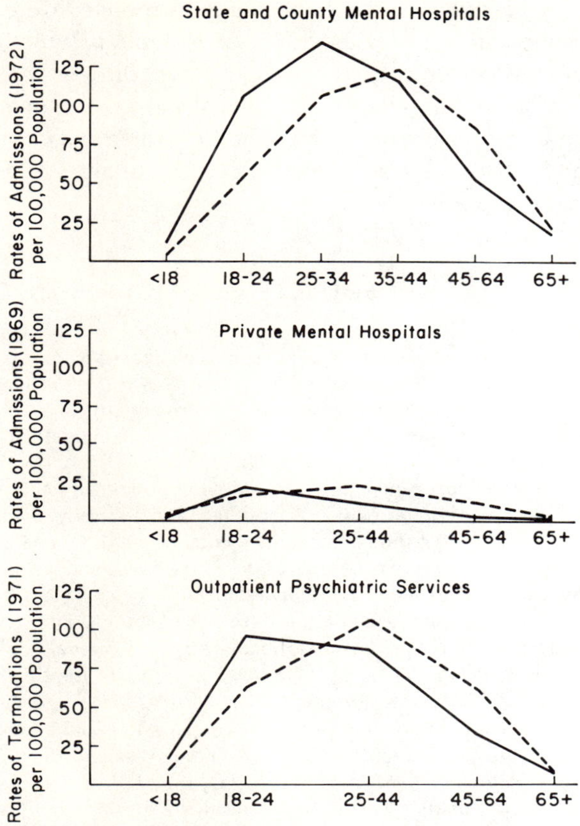

FIGURE 2.7. Utilization rates for schizophrenia at three types of mental health facilities, broken down by age and sex (males—, females---).

which such data were available, male utilization rates for schizophrenia peaked at younger ages and exceeded female utilization rates in the younger age groups; female rates peaked somewhat later and exceeded male rates in the older age groups. This pattern can be seen clearly in Figure 2.7. At each type of facility, the age trend for schizophrenia for each sex reflects rising rates at the younger ages, peak rates somewhere between the age group 18–24 and 25–44, with the rate declining thereafter, reaching a low point in the oldest age group.

CONCLUSION

After reviewing evidence of sex and age differences in the diagnoses made when patients are treated for mental health problems, it can be seen that while, as shown in Chapter 1, overall sex differences in utilization rates were negligible, sex differences in diagnoses received were remarkably consistent amongst all kinds of facilities. As to the four types of disorders singled out for consideration, men had higher rates of treatment for alcohol and drug disorders, while women dramatically exceeded men in rates of diagnosed depressive disorders. Schizophrenia was a major diagnosis for both sexes, and both males and females had essentially identical rates of treatment for schizophrenia.

SOURCES FOR FIGURES IN CHAPTER 2

Figure 2.1. (Distribution in private mental hospitals was based on the National Institute of Mental Health publication, *Private Mental Hospitals, 1969–1970* Washington, D.C.: U.S. Government Printing Office; Distribution in outpatient psychiatric services was based on Table 18 of the National Institute of Mental Health publication, *Outpatient Psychiatric Services, 1971–1972 Washington, D.C.: U.S. Government Printing Office.* [As the National Institute of Mental Health source indicates, "This table excludes terminations from outpatient psychiatric services affiliated with VA hospitals and federally funded community health centers."]; Distribution in state and county mental hospitals was based on Tables 1A and 1C in Meyer, N. G., *Age, sex and color variations in the diagnostic distribution of admissions to inpatient services of state and county mental hospitals, United States, 1972* Washington, D.C.: U.S. Government Printing, Office; Distribution in community mental health centers was based in Table 43 of the National Institute of Mental Health publication, *Provisional Data on Federally Funded Community Mental Health Centers, 1973–1974* Washington, D.C.: U.S. Government Printing Office; Distribution in general hospital inpatient psychiatric units was based on numbers reported in Table B and E of the National Institute of Mental Health publication, Taube, C. A., *Primary diagnosis of discharges from general hospital psychiatric inpatient units* Washington, D.C.: U.S. Government Printing Office. Population statistics for 1971 were used in the calculations of rates. [As the source indicates, "These data are derived from a sample survey of discharges during the month of February 1971. Estimates shown . . . represent a year's discharges centering on this month, e.g., September 1970–August 1971."])

Figure 2.3. (Rates at private mental hospitals based on Table 4 of the National Institute of Mental Health publication, *Private mental hospitals, 1969–1970 Washington, D.C.: U.S. Government Printing Office.* [As the source indicates, numbers include "estimates for hospitals that did not report."]; Rates at outpatient psychiatric services are based on Table 18 of the National Institute of Mental Health publication, *Outpatient psychiatric services, 1971–1972. Washington, D.C.: U.S. Government Printing Office* [As the National Institute of Mental Health sources indicate, "This table excludes terminations from outpatient psychiatric services affiliated with VA hospitals and federally funded community mental health centers."])

Figure 2.5. (Rates at state and county mental hospitals are based on Table 5 of the National Institute of Mental Health publication, Redick, R. W., *Utilization of psychiatric facilities by persons diagnosed with depressive disorders*; Washington, D.C.: U.S. Government Printing Office; For rates at private mental hospitals: See Figure 2.3 legend. Outpatient psychiatric services: see state and county, this legend.)

Figure 2.7 (Private mental hospitals: See Figure 2.3 legend; Outpatient psychiatric services: See Figure 2.3 legend; State and county: See definition of *depressive disorders* in Figure 2.1 legend.)

Chapter 3

COMMUNITY SURVEYS: SEX DIFFERENCES IN MENTAL ILLNESS

Noreen Goldman
Renee Ravid

The utilization data analyzed in the previous chapters indicate the *extent* of treatment, not the *need* for treatment; the data on admissions and additions to mental health facilities can tell us which sex is receiving more medical attention, not which sex is more prone to mental illness. Thus, the question remains: Which sex, or which demographic group within each sex, runs the greater risk of incurring mental illness?

The epidemiological survey attempts to find "true" prevalence by studying a random sample of a noninstitutional population of a community to determine the mental status of the respondents to a questionnaire or interview. Theoretically, the epidemiological survey canvasses both the mentally ill who have received professional help and those who have not.

This chapter will review 22 such surveys that focus on sex differences in mental illness. We have highlighted those studies conducted during the last 15 years and excluded foreign studies to avoid the problems involved with use of international guidelines of psychological evaluation.

The review will question the validity of estimates of "true" prevalence and of recent findings on the interaction between demographic variables (e.g., sex, age, marital status) and mental illness. Let us first examine some previous futile attempts to estimate true prevalence of mental illness as opposed to treatment prevalence.

ISBN 0-12-310850-0

TRUE PREVALENCE: FACT OR FICTION

In their review of epidemiological surveys of mental illness, Dohrenwend and Dohrenwend (1969) note with chagrin that the findings of these surveys would seem to indicate that the prevalence of mental illness ranges from less than 1% to more than 64%, depending on the locale. In their summary of 11 community surveys, Plunkett and Gordon found an equally egregious variation in prevalence: from 16.7 per 1000 to 333 per 1000 (Manis, Brawer, Hunt, & Kercher, 1964). This gross inconsistency, however, reflects not the true prevalence of mental illness, but rather the bias of the investigator, as Manis *et al.* (1964) and others illustrate.

Methodology varies considerably from study to study. Different data-gathering techniques—interviews, questionnaires, clinical evaluations—are used by different researchers. Bias in the assessment of the data is compounded by the professional orientation of the psychiatrist, psychologist, general practitioner, nurse, or social worker who is evaluating the study. Perhaps the factors most influential in creating diversity in methodologies are the disparate criteria for defining mental illness, an absence of standardized scales for detecting mental illness, and a lack of consensus as to how these scales are to be read. Therefore, we must appraise the findings on prevalence in light of the symptomatology under study, the instrument of detection (scale or interview), and the location of the decisive cutoff point on the continuum of mental health to mental illness.

The Dohrenwends (1969) found that "clinical judgment was the tool relied upon for case identification in almost all of the studies [p. 170]" of their review, and that these studies did not usually report in detail "the information available to the judge nor the criteria on which the diagnoses were based [p. 99]"; rather, the "validity of the results is assumed to be implicit in the diagnostic process, a dubious assumption in light of World War II experience with psychiatric screening [p. 170]."

The problem of validity is no less relevant to studies using structured questionnaires than to interviews in which the evaluation of the mental status of the interviewee is dependent upon the erring eye of the beholder. For instance, the 22-item Midtown Scale, developed in the course of the Midtown Manhattan Study (Srole, Langner, Michael, Opler, & Rennie 1962), is a common tool in mental illness detection. In several unrelated studies of prevalence using this scale, the cutoff point varies. Scores ranging from 4 to 10 of the 22 symptoms selected to distinguish between a patient group and a "known well group" in the original Midtown study were used as cutoff points: 10 symptoms were used in Kalamazoo (Manis *et al.*, 1964), 7 in a Plains state (Meile & Haese, 1969), 4 in New Hampshire (Phillips, 1966) and 4 in New York City (Haberman, 1970). Obviously, in these studies prevalence is a function of the cutoff point. As Manis *et al.* (1964) note in connection with the Midtown Manhattan, Baltimore (Commission on Chronic Illness [1957]), and Kalamazoo Studies, the discrepancies in reported prevalence rates "arise primarily from lack of agreement . . . in the criteria used to establish the cutting point between the sick and well [p. 89]."

Dohrenwend and Dohrenwend (1974) find that with a few possible exceptions, there is little evidence of content validity, criterion-oriented validity, or construct validity in any of the epidemiological studies they review (p. 426). We may therefore conclude that due to methodological variations in community surveys, estimates of true prevalence are unreliable.

SEX DIFFERENCES IN MENTAL ILLNESS: DIFFERENT RATES FOR DIFFERENT DIAGNOSES?

Variations in methodology are likely to influence estimates of interactions between demographic variables and mental illness, but most likely these effects will be less than those on estimates of true prevalence. For example, the scale used in a particular study may greatly overestimate or underestimate the prevalence of mental illness, but it may do so equally for males and for females. In such a case, the calculation of the relative rates of mental illness for males and females remains relatively accurate. The more the findings recur across studies, the more confident we may be of their correctness, if we confine our conclusions to the specific form of mental illness to which the findings relate.

Gove and Tudor (1973), Weissman and Klerman (1976), and Dohrenwend and Dohrenwend (1969, 1974) each compiled reviews of community surveys investigating sex differences in one or more types of mental illness. Their findings appear in Tables 3.1-3.7. The results of our review are briefly summarized in Table 3.8.

All 19 of the United States and foreign community studies reported by Gove and Tudor (1973) show a higher percentage of mentally ill females than males. The nature of the mental illness (e.g., mental impairment, anxiety) varies among surveys in the review, but always falls in the diagnostic categories of neurotic disorders and functional psychoses. Of the 14 United States and foreign community surveys on depression investigated by Weissman and Klerman (1976), all except one again report higher rates of mental illness among women. Our findings also seem to reinforce the impression that the prevalence of those mental illnesses studied in recent years is higher among women than among men. Of the 22 studies we in-

TABLE 3.1
Percentage of Men and Women Found to Be Mentally Ill in Community Surveys

SOURCE	MALE	FEMALE	SAMPLE SIZE
	Rates based solely on responses to structured interview		
Martin, Brotherston, and Chave (1957, p. 200)	25	Over 40	750
Phillips and Segal (1969, p. 61)	21.2	35.5	278
Phillips (1966)	21	34	600
Bradburn and Caplovitz (1965, p. 30)	31	54	2006
Tauss (1967, p. 122)	18.4	38.0	707
Taylor and Chave (1964, p. 50)	22	43	422
Gurin, Veroff, and Feld (1960, p. 189)[a]	22	40	2460
Haberman (1969):			
Washington Heights	18.2	25.3	1865
New York City	14.9	33.3	706
Hare and Shaw (1965, p. 25):			
New Adam	15.6	22.9	1015
Old Bute	13.1	26.3	924
Public Health Service (1970, p. 27)[b]	14.9	34.2	6672
Bradburn (1969, p. 119)[c]	20.3	38.9	2379
Meile and Haese (1969, p. 239)	....	*d*	5498
	Rates based on clinical evaluation (psychosis and neurosis)		
Pasamanick *et al.* (1959, p. 188)	4.2	7.1	809
Primrose (1962, pp. 18–24)[e]	4.7	14.7	1701
Essen-Möller (1956, pp. 148–49)	1.7	3.7	2550
Hagnell (1966, pp. 99–103)[e,f]	6.0	15.6	2550
	Rates based on several sources[g] (psychosis and neurosis)		
Leighton *et al.* (1963, pp. 265–67)	45	66	1010

SOURCE: Adapted from Gove, W., and Tudor, J., Adult Sex Roles and Mental Illness, *American Journal of Sociology*, 1973, *78*, 819. (Reprinted with permission.)

a Gurin *et al.* (1960) present their data along four symptom factors—psychological anxiety, physical health, immobilization, and physical anxiety. The figures presented refer to a score of 5 or more on the psychological anxiety factor. Women also scored higher than men on the other three factors.

b Rate indicates persons with three or more symptoms.

c Rates of persons high on symptoms of anxiety.

d 2.5 times male rate.

e Study involved the complete survey of an entire community and excludes psychosis due to organic disorder.

f Rates for neurosis calculated by authors from data on pp. 99–102. (Child neurosis was not considered when calculating the rates.)

g Rates combine psychosis and neurosis and are based on interviews, observations of interviewer, hospital and other institutional records, impressions of physicians in contact with respondent, and impressions of community informants.

TABLE 3.2
Sex Differences in Depression: Community Surveys

PLACE AND TIME	SEX RATIOS (FEMALE:MALE)	REFERENCE
In United States		
Brooklyn and Queens. New York 1960	Women were more depressed	Benfari *et al.* (1972)
Baltimore, Maryland 1968	1.6:1 (Includes wives of blue-collar workers only.)	Siassi *et al.* (1974)
Northern Florida 1968	1.8:1	Schwab *et al.* 1973)
Carroll County, Maryland 1968	Women were more nervous, helpless, anxious.	Hogarty & Katz (1971)
New Haven, Connecticut 1969	2:1 (Suicidal feelings)	Paykel *et al.* (1974)
St. Louis Missouri 1968–1969	No significant sex differences in depression in bereaved spouse.	Clayton *et al.* (1972)
New York, New York 20-Year Period	More referrals for minor depression in female employees in one company.	Hinkle *et al.* (1960)
Outside United States		
Iceland 1910–1957	1.6:1 (All depressions)	Juel-Neilsen *et al.* (1961)
Samso, Denmark 1960	3.5:1 (All depressions)	Sorenson & Stromgren (1961)
Ghiraz, Iran 1964	3.6:1 ($N = 23$)	Bash & Bash-Liechti (1969; 1974)
Lucknow, India 1969–1971	2:1	Sethi (1974)
Herfordshire, England 1949–1954	2.4:1	Martin, *et al.* (1957)
Agra, India (Time not indicated)	1.6:1 (Manic depression)	Dube & Kumar (1973)
Aarhus County, Denmark 1960–1964	1.6:1 (Manic depression) 3.8:1 (Psychogenic depression) 2.9:1 (Neurotic depression)	Weeke *et al.* (1975)

SOURCE: From Table 2 of a study by Weissman, M. M., & Klerman, G. L. *Archives of General Psychiatry*, 1977, *34*, 98–111.

vestigated, 18 compare the overall male and female prevalence rates for some type of mental illness. Sixteen studies point to higher rates for females; 2 report no sex differences. Not one study finds the overall rate of mental illness to be higher for males than females.

However, this implication of greater female vulnerability to mental illness requires a closer examination of the *type* of mental illness being studied, as is reflected in the Dohrenwends' (1969, 1974) explanation of the sex differences seen in community surveys. In their 1969 review of United

TABLE 3.3
Rates of Psychological Disorder Reported for Males and Females

RATE FOR MALES HIGHER (%)				RATE FOR FEMALES HIGHER (%)			
MALE	FEMALE	D	AUTHOR(S)	MALE	FEMALE	D	AUTHOR(S)
1.1[a]	1.0[a]	.1	Kaila, Study II (1942)	1.89[a]	1.91[a]	.02	Rosanoff (1917)
1.3[a]	1.2[a]	.1	Kaila, Study I (1942)	3.0[a]	3.1[a]	.1	Tsuwaga *et al* (1942)
11.9	11.8	.1	Fremming (1951)	1.5[a]	2.0[a]	.5	Lemkau *et al.* (1942)
1.4[a]	1.2[a]	.2	Brugger (1931)	2.0[a]	2.7[a]	.7	Eaton & Weil (1955)
1.0[a]	0.6[a]	.4	Uchimara *et al.* (1940)	1.6[a]	3.3[a]	1.7	Dube (1968)
2.8	1.9	.9	Cohen *et al* (1939)	22.1	24.0	1.9	Bellin & Hardt (1958)
3.4[a]	2.0[a]	1.4	Akimoto *et al.* (1942)	12.3	14.9	2.6	Essen-Möller (1956)
7.9	6.0	1.9	Roth & Luton (1943)	27.2	30.0	2.8	Helgason (1964)
4.5[a]	2.5[a]	2.0	Brugger (1937)	20.6	26.0	5.4	Bremer (1951)
41.8[a]	38.9[a]	2.9	A. H. Leighton *et al.* (1963)	10.0[a]	16.2[a]	6.2	Primrose (1962)
9.0[a]	6.0[a]	3.0	Brugger (1933)	6.0	12.3	6.3	Pasamanick *et al.* (1959)
14.0[a]	9.6[a]	4.4	Gillis *et al.* (1965)	11.3	20.4	9.1	Hagnell (1966a)
				22.6	32.2	9.6	Phillips (1966)
				8.6[a]	20.1[a]	11.5	Strotzka *et al.* (1966)
				12.9[a]	27.5[a]	14.6	Hare & Shaw (1965)
				47.0	65.0	18.0	D. C. Leighton *et al.*,[b] (1963)
				22.0	43.0	21.0	Taylor & Chave[c] (1964)
				51.8[a]	75.2[a]	23.4	Llewellyn-Thomas (1960)

SOURCE: Adapted from B. Dohrenwend, and B. S. Dohrenwend, *Social Status and Psychological Disorder.* New York: Wiley, 1969. p. 15. (Reprinted with permission.)

[a] Calculated by B. S. Dohrenwend.

[b] Results reported in A. H. Leighton *et al.* (1963, p. 149).

[c] Based on survey data without supplementary physicians' reports included in total rate.

TABLE 3.4
Minimum and Maximum Rates of Psychosis Reported According to Sex

RATE FOR MALES HIGHER (%)				RATE FOR FEMALES HIGHER (%)				RATE FOR MALES AND FEMALES EQUAL (%)			
MALE	FEMALE	D	AUTHOR(S)	MALE	FEMALE	D	AUTHOR(S)	MALE	FEMALE	D	AUTHOR(S)
.252[a]	.247[a]	.005	Brugger[b] (1937)	.90[a]	.91[a]	.01	Cohen & Fairbank (1938)	1.60	1.60	.00	Gillis *et al.*[e] (1965)
.45[a]	.40[a]	.05	Brugger[b] (1933)	.34[a]	.35[a]	.01	Dube (1968)				
.70	.63	.07	Lemkau *et al.* (1942)	.44[a]	.46[a]	.02	Kaila, Study I,[b] (1942)				
.57[a]	.44[a]	.13	Akimoto *et al.*[b,c] (1942)	.23[a]	.27[a]	.04	Brugger[b] (1931)				
				.53[a]	.70[a]	.17	Eaton & Weil[g] (1955)				
.51[a]	.22[a]	.29	Tsuwaga *et al.*[b] (1942)	1.7	1.9	.2	Hare & Shaw New Adam (1965)				
.60	.30	.30	Pasamanick *et al.* (1959)	.85[a]	1.48[a]	.63	Primrose (1962)				
.91[a]	.57[a]	.34	Bremer[b] (1951)	.23[a]	.97[a]	.74	Essen-Möller (1956)				
2	1	1	A. H. Leighton *et al.*[d,e] (1963)	1	2	1	D. C. Leighton *et al.*[e] (1963)				
4.6	3.0	1.6	Hare & Shaw (Old Bute) (1965)	1.84[a]	3.63[a]	1.79	Fremming[b,g] (1951)				
....	....	....	Gnat *et al.*[a] 1964	3.99[a]	6.15[a]	2.16	Helgason[b,g] (1964)				

SOURCE: From B. Dohrenwend and B. S. Dohrenwend, *Social Status and Psychological Disorder.* New York: Wiley, 1969. P. 25. (Reprinted with permission.)

[a] Calculated by B. S. Dohrenwend.

[b] Functional psychoses only.

[c] Inconsistencies in age and sex distribution of sample reconciled by making smallest possible number of changes in order to correct what appear to be printer's errors.

[d] Villages only; no psychoses reported in city sample.

[e] Figures are given for "symptom patterns" which may or may not be "cases."

[f] Rates by sex are not given, but text states, "The incidence of mental disorders is greater among women than among men. This applies to all psychiatric disturbances with the exception of psychosis . . . [p. 6]."

[g] Rates for lifetime morbidity.

TABLE 3.5

Minimum and Maximum Rates for Neurosis Reported According to Sex

Rate for Males Higher (%)				Rate for Females Higher (%)			
MALE	FEMALE	D	AUTHOR(S)	MALE	FEMALE	D	AUTHOR(S)
.14[a]	.11[a]	.03	Brugger (1931)	.22[a]	.26[a]	.04	Brugger (1933)
.36[a]	.15[a]	.21	Akimoto *et al.*[b] (1942)	.20	.42	.22	Lemkau *et al.* (1942)
				.00	.37[a]	.37	Tsuwaga *et al.* (1942)
81	69	12	A. H. Leighton *et al.* (city)[c] (1963)	1.07[a]	1.86[a]	.79	Essen-Möller (1956)
				1.46[a]	2.34[a]	.88	Fremming[d] (1951)
76	64	12	A. H. Leighton *et al.* (villages)[c] (1963)	.30[a]	1.31[a]	1.01	Eaton & Weil[d] (1955)
				.40[a]	2.28[a]	1.88	Dube (1968)
				3.56	6.80	3.24	Pasamanick *et al.* (1959)
				3.2	6.9	3.7	Hagnell (1959)
				3.6	8.0	4.4	Hare & Shaw (New Adam) (1965)
				5.6	10.5	4.9	Hare & Shaw (Old Bute) (1965)
				2.91	8.30	5.39	Bremer (1951)
				24.40[a]	36.80[a]	12.40	Gillis *et al.*[c] (1965)
				6.85[a]	13.95[a]	7.10	Helgason[d] (1964)
				4.4	13.6	9.2	Primrose (1962)
				44	64	20	D. C. Leighton *et al.*[c] (1963)
				......	......	......	Gnat *et al.*[e] (1964)

Source: From B. Dohrenwend and B. S. Dohrenwend, *Social Status and Psychological Disorder.* New York: Wiley, 1969. P. 27. (Reprinted with permission.)

[a] Calculated by B. S. Dohrenwend.

[b] Inconsistencies in age and sex distribution of sample reconciled by making smallest possible number of changes in order to correct what appear to be printer's errors.

[c] Figures are given for "symptom patterns" which may or may not be "cases."

[d] Rates for lifetime morbidity.

[e] Rates by sex are not given, but text states, "The incidence of mental disorders is greater among women than among men. This applies to all psychiatric disturbances with the exception of psychosis, alcoholism and mental disorders following brain injury (p. 6)."

TABLE 3.6

Minimum and Maximum Rates of Personality Disorder Reported According to Sex

Rate for Males Higher (%)				Rate for Females Higher (%)			
MALE	FEMALE	D	AUTHOR(S)	MALE	FEMALE	D	AUTHOR(S)
.11[a]	.01[a]	.10	Brugger (1931)	.046[a]	.047[a]	.001	Eaton & Weil[c] (1955)
.40[a]	.11[a]	.29	Akimoto *et al.*[b] (1942)	9.27	9.43	.16	Bremer (1951)
				.73[a]	.97[a]	.24	Tsuwaga *et al.* (1942)
.63[a]	.12[a]	.51	Brugger (1937)	4.5	6.5	2.0	Hare & Shaw (New Adam) (1965)
10.0	9.3	.7	Hare & Shaw (Old Bute) (1965)				
1.08[a]	.18[a]	.90	Brugger (1933)				
5.02[a]	4.09[a]	.93	Helgason[c] (1964)				
5.85[a]	2.94[a]	2.91	Fremming[c] (1951)				
4.73[a]	1.14[a]	3.59	Primrose (1962)				
5.20[a]	.00	5.20	Gillis *et al.*[d,f] (1965)				
18[a]	11[a]	7	D. C. Leighton *et al.*[d,e] (1963)				
9.15[a]	1.62[a]	7.53	Essen-Möller (1956)				
13[a]	5[a]	8	A. H. Leighton *et al.*[d,f] (1963)				
......	......	......	Gnat *et al.*[g] (1964)				

SOURCE: From B. Dohrenwend and B. S. Dohrenwend, *Social Status and Psychological Disorder*. New York: Wiley, 1969. P. 27. (Reprinted with permission.)

[a] Calculated by B. S. Dohrenwend.

[b] Inconsistencies in age and sex distribution reconciled by making smallest possible number of changes in order to correct what appear to be printer's errors.

[c] Rates for lifetime morbidity.

[d] Figures are given for "symptom patterns" which may or may not be "cases."

[e] Personality disorder and sociopathic behavior combined, although these categories are not mutually exclusive, of 128 cases in the two categories, only 10 are classified in both; also, rate for males is higher than for females in each category.

[f] Personality disorder and sociopathic behavior combined, although not mutually exclusive, on the basis of the small overlap in D. C. Leighton *et al.* which provided the procedural base for this study; also, rate for males is higher than for females in each category. Figures are given for "symptom patterns" which may or may not be "cases."

[g] No figures were given, but text stated that males exceeded females on alcoholism while females exceeded males on behavior disorders. Since 29 cases of the former and 3 of the latter were given, the presumption is that males exceed females in the two categories combined.

TABLE 3.7
Comparison of Male and Female Rates of Different Types of Psychopathology Reported in European and North American Studies According to Rural and Urban Study Sites and Date of Publication

		STUDY SITE					
		RURAL		URBAN		MIXED	
		NUMBER OF STUDIES IN WHICH RATE IS HIGHER FOR:					
DATE OF PUBLICATION	TYPE OF PSYCHOPATHOLOGY	MALES	FEMALES	MALES	FEMALES	MALES	FEMALES
Before 1950	All	4	1	1	1	2	0
	Psychosis	2	1	1	1	0	1
	Neurosis	1	1	0	1	–	–
	Personality disorder	3	0	–	–	–	–
1950 or After	All	1	13	0	5	–	–
	Psychosis	1	6	3	1	–	–
	Neurosis	0	9	0	4	–	–
	Personality disorder	5	2	2	1	–	–

SOURCE: From B. Dohrenwend and B. S. Dohrenwend, Social and Cultural Influences on Psychopathology. *Annual Review of Psychology,* 1974, *25,* 438. (Reprinted with permission.)

States and foreign studies, they report that for *overall psychological disorder,* 18 studies find higher rates for women and 12 find higher rates for men (Table 3.3). Thus, here there are no overwhelming sex differences. But when studies are broken down by type of mental illness, different patterns emerge, as seen in Tables 3.4, 3.5, and 3.6. Whereas no marked sex difference is evident for psychoses studies, females have higher rates in 17 out of 21 studies on neuroses while males have higher rates in 13 of the 17 studies on personality disorders. Curiously, Table 3.7 shows that studies prior to 1950 reveal a higher rate of mental illness for men in 7 out of 9 studies: studies conducted after 1950 reveal a higher rate for women—18 out of 19 studies. The Dohrenwends (1974) attribute this disturbing increase in mental illness among women to the type of study and scale used in later surveys [p. 439]. Of course, it is possible that there has been a real change over time in the symptomatology experienced by each sex. But the Dohrenwends suggest that scales such as the 22-item Midtown Scale, used in over 30% of the 22 studies of our review, detect symptoms of neurotic behavior rather than symptoms of psychoses or personality disorders.

As Table 3.8 shows, *no* study in our review focuses on symptoms of personality disorder; few are constructed to detect psychoses. Many sift out allied types of mental illness. Others detect forms of mental duress that perhaps should not be classified as mental illness at all, such as anxiety, maladjustment, and unhappiness.

TABLE 3.8
United States Community Surveys on Sex Differences in Mental Illness

AUTHOR AND PUBLICATION YEAR	DATE OF STUDY	LOCATION OF STUDY	SAMPLE SIZE	TYPE OF MENTAL ILLNESS INVESTIGATED	SUMMARY OF MALE–FEMALE DIFFERENCES
Baltimore Study (Commission on Chronic Illness [1957]	1952–1956	Urban Baltimore, Md.	11,574	Mental disorder	Overall, women had a higher prevalence of mental disorder than men (131/1000 versus 84/1000). Sex differences depended on the specific diagnosis
Benfari *et al.* (1972)	early 1960s	Brooklyn and Queens, N.Y.	531	Psychoneurotic behavior	Women obtained higher scores in anxiety–depression and anxiety–vegetative disorders; there were no sex differences in low esteem, withdrawal, and cognitive depression.
Bradburn (1969)	1963–1964	5 samples: 2 in Detroit, Mich., One each in Chicago, Ill., Washington D.C., and a group of large metropolitan areas	2787	Happiness; Anxiety	There were no sex differences in happiness. Women scored higher on the anxiety scale than men (38.9% versus 20.3% with high scores).
Bradburn and Caplovitz (1965)	early 1960s	4 communities in Illinois	2006	Happiness; Anxiety	There were no sex differences in happiness. Women scored higher on the anxiety items than men (54% versus 31% with high scores).
Clayton *et al.* (1972)	1968–1969	St. Louis, Mo.	109 widows and widowers	Depression	Approximately equal percentages of men (33%) and women (36%) were depressed in the first month of bereavement
Dohrenwend (1973)	early 1970s	Washington Heights in New York City, N.Y.	124	Mental impairment (22-item Midtown Scale	Women had higher symptom scores than men.
Eaton and Weil (1955)	1950–1951	Hutterites throughout U.S. and Canada (N. Dakota, S. Dakota, Alberta, Manitoba, Montana, etc.)	8542	Mental disorder (lifetime prevalence)	Psychoneurotics, manic depressives, and psychotics were more common among women than men (male to female sex ratios were 1:4, 5:8, and .77:1 respectively).
Gurin *et al.* (1960)	1957	Entire U.S.	2460	Mental adjustment; Happiness	There were no sex differences in happiness. Women scored higher than men on all 4 symptom factors: psychological anxiety, physical health, immobilization, and physical anxiety.

(continued)

TABLE 3.8 (CONT.)
United States Community Surveys on Sex Differences in Mental Illness

AUTHOR AND PUBLICATION YEAR	DATE OF STUDY	LOCATION OF STUDY	SAMPLE SIZE	TYPE OF MENTAL ILLNESS INVESTIGATED	SUMMARY OF MALE–FEMALE DIFFERENCES
Haberman (1970)	early 1960s	Washington Heights in New York City, and the 5 boroughs of New York City, N.Y.	1865 in Washington Heights; 706 in New York City	Mental impairment (22-item Midtown Scale)	Women had higher rates of impairment than men: 25.3% of women versus 18.2% of men had 4 or more symptoms in Washington Heights; 33.3% of women versus 14.9% of men had 4 or more symptoms in New York City.
Hogarty and Katz (1971)	1968	Carroll County, Md.	450	Adjustment and social behavior (Katz Adjustment Scale)	Women had significantly higher mean scores on nervousness, helplessness, and anxiety. Men did not score higher on any of the symptom clusters.
Knupfer *et al.* (1966)	1962	San Francisco, Calif.	979	Overall happiness; Adjustment	More single men (21%) were unhappy than single women (12%) and than married men (7%). Married women indicated more unhappiness than married men (10% versus 7%)
Markush and Favero (1974)	1972	Washington County, Md. and Kansas City, Mo.	1240 in W.C.; 889 in K.C.	Depression (CES-D Scale); Mental impairment (22-item Midtown Scale)	Women had higher scores than men on both the CES-D Scale and the 22-item scale. On the CES-D Scale, 23% of women vs. 13% of men scored high in W.C. and 25% of women versus 17% of men scored high in K.C. On the Midtown Scale, 14% of women versus 6% of men had 4 or more symptoms in W.C. and 15% of women versus 9% of men had 4 or more symptoms in K.C.
Meile and Haese (1969)		3 communities in a plains state	6018	Mental impairment (22-item Midtown Scale)	Females were approximately 2 1/2 times as likely as males to report symptoms of mental stress.

Pearlin (1975)	1972	Chicago, Ill.	2300	Depression (11-Symptom Scale)	Women indicated more depression than men.
Pearlin and Johnson (1975)		Chicago, Ill.	2300	Depression	For both sexes, the married were the least disposed to depression and the formerly married the most. (Results were not presented separately for the sexes.)
Phillips (1966)		New Hampshire	600	Mental impairment (22-item Midtown Scale)	More women than men had high scores on the 22-item scale: 32.2% of women versus 22.6% of men had 4 or more symptoms.
Phillips and Segal (1969)	1964–1965	Lebanon, N.H.	302	Mental impairment (22-item Midtown Scale and four subindices)	Women scored considerably higher than men on the 22-item scale on the psychological index, and on the psychophysiological index: 35.5% of women versus 21.2% of men had 4 or more symptoms. Men scored somewhat higher than women on the physiological and the "ambiguous" index.
Radloff (1975)		Kansas City, Mo., and Washington County, Md.	1159 in K.C.; 1670 in W.C.	Depression (CES-D Scale)	In the total sample, women were more depressed than men. Sex differences interacted significantly with marital status.
Schwab *et al.* (1968)		Medical inpatients at a hospital in Florida	153	Depression	Women showed more depression than men (25% of women versus 16% of men were depressed).
Schwab *et al.* (1973)	1968	County in U.S. Southeast	318	Social psychiatric impairment	Among blacks there were no sex differences, but 19% fewer of the white men than the white women were impaired.
Siassi *et al.* (1974)	1968	General Motors plant, Baltimore, Md.	888	Loneliness; Depression	Wives felt more lonely and depressed than their blue-collar husbands.
Srole *et al.* (1962)	early 1950s	Midtown Manhattan, N.Y.	1660	Mental impairment (22-item Midtown Scale)	No statistically significant sex differences occurred in any age group. The interaction between sex differences and marital status was significant, however.

Assessments based on studies implementing the 22-item Midtown Scale and similar scales should therefore be more modest in scope. To argue that more women than men become mentally ill is to reduce appreciably the definition of mental illness to certain types of neuroses. As the Dohrenwends (1974) emphasize in discussing the Gove and Tudor review (1973):

> They [Gove and Tudor] made a decision about the definition of psychopathology that badly compromised their treatment of the question. They defined "mental illness" as consisting of neurotic disorders and functional psychoses if the studies provided data in the form of diagnoses, or as "personal discomfit" as indicated by measures of subjective distress and anxiety if the studies provided data in the form of symptom scores only. In doing so, they combined disparate types of psychopathology and they excluded a major diagnostic category, personality disorder [p. 437].

If certain types of neuroses are female modes of expressing distress, we should balance studies focusing on these neuroses with studies that diagnose other forms of mental illness, including psychoses and personality disorders, in order to arrive at estimates of the true prevalence of mental illness for each sex.

Several of the studies in our review do, in fact, analyze their data separately for different diagnoses. Their findings corroborate the Dohrenwends' contention that the interaction between sex and mental illness depends on the specific form of mental illness considered. Knupfer, Clark, and Room (1966) report that women experience more symptoms of anxiety, worry, and phobias than men, whereas men manifest more severe neurotic symptoms than women. Using the 22-item Midtown Scale and 4 subindices based on this scale, Phillips and Segal (1969) note that women score higher than men on the Midtown Scale, the psychological index, and the psychophysiological index, while men score somewhat higher on the physiological index and on the ambiguous index (which consists of degrees of organic illness). The Baltimore Study (Commission on Chronic Illness [1957]) reports that women score higher for psychoneuroses and for psychophysiologic, autonomic, and visceral disorders, but that men score higher than women for other mental and personality disorders. Benfari, Beiser, Leighton, and Mertens (1972) conclude that females score higher for symptoms of anxiety–depression and anxiety–vegetative disturbance, but that there are no significant sex differences for withdrawal and cognitive depression.

Other investigators have found that females score higher than males for all of the particular diagnoses being studied. Eaton and Weil (1955) conclude that manic depressives, psychotics, and psychoneurotics are more common among women than men; Markush and Favero (1974) find females scoring higher than males on both the Center for Epidemiologic Studies Depression Scale (the CES-D Scale) and on the 22-item Midtown Scale; and Gurin, Veroff, and Feld (1960) report that women score higher than men on all 4 of the symptom factors listed by Gurin *et al.*—psychological anxiety, physical health, immobilization, and physical anxiety.

The bulk of studies during the last decade or two concentrate on neurotic symptomatology, which women appear to run a greater risk of experiencing. But to date, there are insufficient data to pinpoint the specific forms of mental illness for which the female prevalence rate is higher. Some scales, such as the CES-D Scale for depression, do attempt to represent a diagnosis, but many do not. Furthermore, many investigators advise us of the limitations of their scales. Pearlin (1975), for example, issues a common disclaimer for the 11-symptom depression scale developed by Lipman, Rickels, Cori, Derogatis, and Uhlenhuth (1969) and by Derogatis, Lipman, Covi, and Rickels (1971):

> The tone and content of the items define depression as a condition of malaise, apathy, or weary disaffection. It should be emphasized that such items, when used in a survey of a normal population, are not suitable for the identification of clinical depression. They do not necessarily reveal psychiatric "cases," they do not point out those needing psychiatric help, and they do not indicate functional impairment—whether or not people are able to fulfill their social roles in a usual manner. Scores on these measures have no absolute clinical meaning. Their utility lies in their ability to discern an order among people based on the relative degree of depression they express. Because these scales are constructed from the symptoms reported by the patients in a clinical treatment, it can be mistakenly assumed that a high score thus indicates a need for treatment. In field studies using representative samples, these scales are not diagnostic tools and scores are not indicative of whether people need clinical care [p. 186].

Elaborating on this point, the Dohrenwends (1969) differentiate between persistent disorder and situationally specific symptoms:

> It appears, then, that the determinations of psychological disorder made in community studies including our own research in Washington Heights can no longer be accepted at face value. To do so would require acceptance of claims that untreated "cases" in the general populations show the same types of stereotyped and repetitive symptomatology as has been observed in patients over long courses of treatment, without any direct information about the duration of an individual's symptoms over time and in different situational contexts [p. 171].

Other scales and interviews measure mental distress not in terms of clinical diagnoses, but as a more vague mental disability, such as mental impairment, psychiatric impairment, tension, anxiety, or unhappiness. As noted earlier, one wonders why some of these are included under the heading of mental illness.

Thus, as we have seen, current evidence from community surveys supports the conclusion that more females are experiencing the symptoms under study than males. The significance of these symptoms, however, in terms of specific forms of mental illness as opposed to broad classifications, such as mental impairment, has eluded the researchers. Perhaps the real meaning is still to be sorted out from the vast quantities of data. Without consistency in the administering of scales designed to detect specific forms of mental illness, including psychoses and personality disorders, we cannot determine which sex is more susceptible to mental illness over all.

Of course, the question of causation naturally arises. Why do more women than men experience the symptomatology in recent studies? One explanation put forward by Gove and Tudor (1973), is that the ungratifying, restrictive, often demeaning role that married women play in modern Western societies is a source of emotional problems. They argue that generally speaking, the married woman's major societal role—that of housewife—entails frustrating, unstructured, and hardly prestigious chores such as raising children and keeping house. The typical married working woman is discriminated against in the job market, is more committed to supplementing the family income than to furthering a career, and must bear the additional onus of doing the housework.

An opposing explanation offered by Phillips and Segal (1969) is that the disproportionately greater rate of mental illness among women is due not to "real sex differences in frequency of disturbance but rather to man's greater reluctance to admit certain unpleasurable feelings and sensations [p. 69]." It is suggested that "women may be more likely than men to *report* certain acts, behaviors, and feelings that lead to their being categorized as mentally ill [p. 59; emphasis in original]" because "it is more culturally appropriate and acceptable for women to be more expressive about their difficulties [p. 59]."

SEX AND OTHER DEMOGRAPHIC VARIABLES

Marital Status

As would be expected, certain other demographic variables play a part in the interaction between sex and mental illness. Of the seven demographic variables investigated in this review—marital status, age, race, parental status, education, income, and employment status—marital status is most strikingly related to mental illness. In an examination of 17 community and utilization studies, Gove (1972) finds that in *all* of the studies married women have higher rates of mental illness (defined differently in the various studies) than married men; in 11 out of 15 studies, single men have higher rates than single women. Gove's analysis (1972) of studies of the formerly married yields somewhat less consistent results. Most of the studies show that men have higher rates of mental illness than women for both the divorced and widowed categories.

The findings of our review are similar but not as clearcut. The most consistent finding is that single men are more "maladjusted," "mentally impaired," or depressed than single women. This is the result reported by Knupfer, *et al.* (1966), Bradburn and Caplovitz (1965), Radloff (1975), Srole *et al.* (1962), and Gurin *et al.* (1960). In no study are single women shown as more prone to mental illness than single men. Bradburn (1969) finds single men and single women to be equally "happy," or "unhappy." Results for the currently married are not as clear. Radloff (1975) reports that married women are more depressed than married men; Knupfer *et al.* (1966) find that married women evince more distress and anxiety symptoms than married men; and finally, Srole *et al.* (1962) discern no difference in mental impairment between married men and women.

There is even less consistency in findings on the divorced, separated, and widowed. Bradburn (1969) and Bradburn and Caplovitz (1965) report that previously married men are less happy than previously married women; Radloff (1975) finds divorced or separated women more depressed than men of this category; and Gurin *et al.* (1960) also note that divorced or separated women are more poorly adjusted than men. But, Srole *et al.* (1962) find no significant sex difference between the widowed and no significant sex difference between the divorced; Clayton, Halkas, and Maurice (1972) confirm this latter finding of no sex difference in depression rates of the widowed. As Gove (1972) notes, for both sexes, rates for the divorced or separated and widowed are higher than those for the married in almost all studies. This finding is supported by surveys conducted by Pearlin and Johnson (1975), Bradburn (1969), Bradburn and Caplovitz (1965), Srole *et al.* (1962), and Gurin *et al.* (1960).

To date, studies suggest that single men are more maladjusted than married men (e.g., Knupfer *et al.*, 1966; Srole *et al.*, 1962), but that there is often no significant difference in rates of mental illness of single and married women. Radloff's study (1975) supports this finding. Barring unemployment, the evidence strongly suggests that marriage is better for men; that is, married men are less depressed than single men, and less depressed than married women. However, we should refrain from deducing causation merely because there is a correlation between variables. It is misleading to imply that he who marries is less likely to be depressed. If a selection factor is operating here, it may rather be that he who is less depressed is more likely to marry.

Age

Findings on the relationship between sex, age, and mental illness vary considerably from study to study. Nevertheless, the data warrant our suggesting that, in general, the age patterns of mental illness are similar for men and women. Radloff (1975) and Markush and Favero (1974) find that scores on the CES-D Scale decrease with age for both sexes. On the 22-item Midtown Scale, however, Markush and Favero find no consistent age pattern. Benfari *et al.* (1972) conclude that age patterns vary substantially with the type of symptom factor under consideration. The age patterns are similar for both sexes for topically oriented depression, esteem, and self-confidence. However, the patterns for the symptom factors of physiological anxiety, physiological process disturbance, and mixed anxiety–depression vary according to sex, with male and female scores peaking at different ages. Gurin *et al.* (1960) find that for both sexes, scores on the psychological anxiety and physical anxiety factors generally increase with age, but that this tendency is more pronounced among women. Finally, Schwab, Brown and Holzer (1968) note a different age pattern of depression for males than for females, with scores for males peaking at an older age.

Race

Only two of the studies in our review consider racial breakdowns by sex. Both suggest that sex differences in mental illness may not be identical for blacks and whites. As reported by Markush and Favero (1974), on the 22-item Midtown Scale administered in Kansas City, white women have higher scores than white men, yet there is no significant sex difference amongst blacks. Again, in the study of a Southeast county made by Schwab, McGinnis, and Warheit (1973), a significantly lower percentage of white men than white women is rated mentally impaired, while there is no sex difference in rates of impairment among blacks.

When comparing the two races as a whole, without regard to sex, the Markush and Favero study (1974) reports the same percentage of high scores on the CES-D Scale and the Midtown Scale for both races. In reviewing another study, however, Schwab *et al.* (1973) find blacks to be more impaired than whites.

Miscellaneous Demographic Factors

The relationship between sex differences and other demographic variables, such as education, income, parental status, and employment status, has not been studied extensively. Conclusions, based on only two or three studies for each variable, are at best tentative.

In their analysis of true prevalence, the Dohrenwends (1974) point out that the most consistent result reported is an inverse relationship between overall rates of psychopathology and social class (p. 439). The findings of Markush and Favero (1974), Radloff (1975), and Pearlin and Johnson (1975) lend credence to this view. According to Radloff and Pearlin and Johnson, for both sexes, the lower the income, the higher the depression scores; according to Markush and Favero and Radloff, for both sexes, the lower the education, the higher the depression scores.

Contrary to popular opinion, children seem to adversely affect the mental health of their parents. Pearlin (1975) finds that the "role disenchantment" for females increases with the number of children at home, and that the younger the child the greater the disenchantment; and according to Radloff (1975), the CES-D Scale shows that the greater the role disenchantment, the greater the depression. To stay on the safe side of the statistics, it seems advisable to have children, but to rear them as quickly as possible. Radloff (1975) shows that both males and females with "empty nests" evince lower depression scores on the CES-D Scale than those with no children or those whose children still live at home.

There seems to be no statistical basis at present to support the hypothesis that working women are less depressed than full-time homemakers. Both Radloff (1975) and Pearlin (1975) find no significant differences between the two groups with regard to depression. Pearlin concludes that for women, it is not the role that matters but the "conditions that are encountered within the roles [p. 188]." Radloff finds that unemployment is the only condition in which married women are less depressed than married men. Bradburn (1969) likewise notes that men not in the labor force are more "unhappy" than women in the same situation.

To sum up, the most vulnerable group in our 22-study review seems to be the formerly married female of low income and low education; for her, the fewer the children at home, the better her mental state. Perhaps the lowest risk group of these studies would be the white married male, employed, earning a high income, and well-educated.

METHODOLOGICAL PROBLEMS

In this review, we have come across several major obstacles in estimating true prevalence and in determining the relative risk of incurring mental illness for various demographic groups. The evaluator of any study is beset with many difficulties in assessing the data at hand although, unfortunately, his evaluations are often presented or accepted as statistical "truths." There are inherent problems in data gathering that distort the true rates, whatever they may be. We will briefly touch on some of the methodological problems of which the reader of a study is frequently unaware.

First, a host of statistical problems often go unacknowledged in the findings of various studies. Nonresponse or refusal rates are sometimes very high (e.g., 58% in Clayton *et al.*, 1972; 34% in Dohrenwend, 1973); some studies do not even mention this problem (e.g., Hogarty & Katz, 1971). Only one study reviewed here—the Baltimore Study (Commission on Chronic Illness [1957])—attempts to assess the potential bias of nonresponse. A small sample size (109 in Clayton *et al.*, 1972; 153 in Schwab *et al.*, 1968; and 128 in Dohrenwend, 1973) can likewise make the validity of the findings questionable. Many studies analyze one variable at a time for its relationships to mental illness, failing to consider the possibility of multiple interactions among demographic variables. Phillips (1966), for instance, analyzes the relationship between marital status and mental illness, but does *not* examine this relationship for each sex. An approach such as this means there is no possibility of determining, for example, that single men are more depressed than married men but that this distinction does not hold true for females. Many studies do not statistically test their findings. Such studies' comparison of one percentage to another without significance testing may be of no particular use when the sample sizes of the groups being compared are extremely unequal, or small. Studies failing to statistically test for significant differences include Phillips (1966), Knupfer *et al.* (1966); Phillips and Segal (1969); Bradburn and Caplovitz (1965); Eaton and Weil (1955); and Markush and Favero (1974). Also, even if the sample is large, statistically significant differences may be very small, and perhaps have no meaning for us (e.g., as seen in Hogarty & Katz, 1971). Finally, authors of several of the studies do not present enough data for the reader to evaluate the results for himself (e.g., Meile & Haese, 1969; Schwab *et al.*, 1973).

In addition to suffering from these statistical problems, some studies fail to recognize the problems linked to constructing and administering the questionnaire. The type of questionnaire is often not fully described in the study (e.g., Schwab *et al.*, 1973), and the criteria used to determine illness may be unclear. The danger of not defining the criteria for mental illness has already been discussed in this chapter. Furthermore, we have reservations about the reliability of a self-administered questionnaire, such as the one used by Bradburn (1969), and about the reliability of secondary sources of data, as, for example, a file, that are not supplemented with a follow-up interview (e.g., Eaton & Weil, 1955).

In our earlier discussion of some of the pitfalls of varying methodologies, we noted that inferences drawn from any study are applicable only to the form of mental illness under study; that certain scales (e.g., the 11-symptom depression scale) pick up symptoms that have been found in patients but are not necessarily indicative of mental illness; and that other scales detect certain types of malaise which seem remote from mental illness (e.g., unhappiness). The Baltimore Study (Commission on Chronic Illness [1957]) underlines this problem in defining and accurately testing for mental illness. It selected a certain fraction of the sample and followed up home interviews with clinical evaluation diagnoses. Less than one-quarter of all conditions diagnosed in clinical examinations corresponded generally to the initial assessment of the household interview!

CONCLUSIONS

Community studies on sex differences in mental illness reported by Gove and Tudor, Weissman and Klerman, and studies in this review point to higher rates of mental illness for females. However, studies in our review that analyze data separately for different diagnoses support the Dohrenwends' contention that sex differences in mental illness may depend upon the diagnosis being tested. More women than men are afflicted with the symptomatology on which the bulk of recent studies concentrate. However, there are insufficient data to pinpoint the specific forms of mental illness for which female rates are greater, and there has been an insufficient number of studies on sex differences for psychoses and personality disorders to determine which sex is more susceptible to mental illness as a whole. In addition, inferences about sex differences in mental illness may be biased by a host of statistical problems linked to constructing and administering questionnaires.

REFERENCES

Akimoto, H., Shimazaki, T., Okada, K., & Hanasiro, S. Demographische und psychiatrische Untersuchung über abgegrenzte Kleinstadtgevölkerung. *Psychiatria et Neurologia Japonica,* 1942, *47,* 351–374.

Bash, K. W., & Bash-Liechti, J. Studies on the epidemiology of neuro-psychiatric disorders among the rural population of the province of Khuzestan, Iran. *Soc Psychiatry*, 1969, *4*, 137–143.

Bash, K. W., & Bash-Liechti, J. Studies on the epidemiology of neuro-psychiatric disorders among the population of the city of Shiraz, Iran. *Soc Psychiatry*, 1974, *9*, 163–171.

Benfari, R. C., Beiser, M., Leighton, A. H., & Mertens, C. Some dimensions of psychoneurotic behavior in an urban sample. *The Journal of Nervous and Mental Diseases*, 1972, *155*(2), 77–90.

Bradburn, N. *The structure of psychological well-being*. Chicago: Aldine, 1969.

Bradburn, N., & Caplovitz, D. *Reports on happiness*. Chicago: Aldine, 1965.

Bremer, J. A social psychiatric investigation of a small community in northern Norway. *Acta Psychiatrica et Neurologica Scandinavica*, 1951, Supplementum 62.

Brugger, C. Versuch einer Geisteskrankanzählung in Thüringen. *Zeitschrift für die gesamte Neurologie und Psychiatrie*, 1931, *133*, 352–390.

Brugger, C. Psychiatrische Ergebnisse emer medizinischen, anthropologischen, und soziologichen Bevölkerunguntersuchung. *Zeitschrift für die gesamte Neurologie und Psychiatrie*, 1933, *146*, 489–524.

Brugger, C. Psychiatrische Bestandaufnahme im Gebeit eines medizinish-anthropologischen Zensus in der Nähe von Rosenheim. *Zeitschrift für die gesamte Neurologie und Psychiatrie*, 1937, *160*, 189–207.

Bellin, S. S., & Hardt, R. H. Marital status and mental disorders among the aged. *American Sociological Review*, 1958, *23*, 155–162.

Clayton, P. J., Halikas, J. A., & Maurice, W. L. The depression of widowhood. *British Journal of Psychiatry*, 1972, *120*, 71–78.

Cohen, B. M., & Fairbank, R. Statistical contributions from the mental hygiene study of the Eastern Health District of Baltimore. II. Psychosis in the Eastern Health District in 1933. *American Journal of Psychiatry*, 1938, *94*, 1377–1395.

Cohen, B. M., Fairbank, R., & Greene, E. Statistical contributions from the Eastern Health District of Baltimore. III. Personality disorder in the Eastern Health District in 1933. *Human Biology*, 1939, *11*, 112–129.

Commission on Chronic Illness. Chronic illness in a large city: The Baltimore study. Cambridge: Harvard University Press, 1957.

Derogatis, L. R., Lipman, R. S., Covi, L., & Rickels, K. Neurotic symptom dimensions. *Archives of General Psychiatry*, 1971, *24*, 454–464.

Dohrenwend, B. P., & Dohrenwend, B. S. *Social status and psychological disorder: A causal inquiry*. New York: John Wiley and Sons, 1969.

Dohrenwend, B. P., & Dohrenwend, B. S. Social and cultural influences on psychopathology. *Annual Review of Psychology*, 1974, *25*, 417–452.

Dohrenwend, B. S. Social status and stressful life events. *Journal of Personality and Social Psychology*, 1973, *28*(2), 225–235.

Dube, K. C. Mental disorder in Agra. *Social Psychiatry*, 1968, *3*, 139–143.

Dube, K. C., & Kumar, N. An epidemiological study of manic-depressive psychosis. *Acta Psychiat Scand.*, 1973, *49*, 691–697.

Eaton, J., & Weil, R. *Culture and mental disorders*. Glencoe, Ill.: Free Press, 1955.

Essen-Möller, E. Individual traits and morbidity in a Swedish rural population. *Acta Psychiatrica et Neurologica Scandinavica*, 1956, Supplementum 100.

Fremming, K. H. *The Expectation of Mental Infirmity in a Sample of the Danish Population*. London: Eugenics Society, 1951.

Gnat, T., Henisz, J., & Sarapata, A. A psychiatric-socio-statistical study of two Polish towns. Paper read at First International Congress of Social Psychiatry, London, August, 1964.

Gillis, L. S., Lewis, J. B., & Slabbert, M. *Psychiatric Disturbance and Alcoholism in the Coloured People of the Cape Peninsula.* Cape Town: University of Cape Town, Department of Psychiatry, 1965.

Gove, W. The relationship between sex roles, mental illness and marital status. *Social Forces,* 1972, *51*(1), 34–44.

Gove, W. R., & Tudor, J. Adult sex roles and mental illness. *American Journal of Sociology,* 1973, *78,* 812–835.

Gurin, G., Veroff, J., & Feld, S. *Americans view their mental health.* New York: Basic Books, 1960.

Haberman, Paul. 1969. "Cross-Survey Analysis of Psychiatric Symptomology: A Corroborative Report on Subgroup Differences." Paper read at annual meeting of the American Sociological Association, San Francisco.

Haberman, P. W. Ethnic differences in psychiatric symptoms reported in community surveys. *Public Health Reports,* 1970, *85*(6), 495–502.

Hagnell, Olle. 1966. *A Prospective Study of the Incidence of Mental Disorder.* Sweden: Berlingska Boktryckeriet.

Hare, E. H., and G. K. Shaw. 1965. *Mental Health on a New Housing Estate.* London: Oxford University Press.

Helgason, T. Epidemiology of mental disorders in Iceland. *Acta Psychiatrica Scandinavica,* 1964, Supplementum 173.

Hinkle, L. E., Redmont, R., Plummer, N., *et al.* II. An explanation of the relation between symptoms, disability, and serious illness in two homogeneous groups of men and women. *Journal of Public Health,* 1960, *50,* 1327–1336.

Hogarty, G. E., & Katz, M. N. Norms of adjustment and social behavior. *Arch Gen Psychiat.,* 1971, *25,* 470–480.

Juel-Nielson, N., Bille, M., Flygenring, J., & Helgason, T. Frequency of depressive states within geographically delimited population groups. *Acta Psychiat. Scand. Suppl.,* 1961, *162*(37), 69–80.

Kaila, J. Uber die Durchschnittshäufigkeit der Geisteskrankheiten und des Schwachsinns in Finnland. *Acta Psychiatrica et Neurologica,* 1942, *17,* 47–67.

Knupfer, G., Clark, W., & Room, R. The mental health of the unmarried. *American Journal of Psychiatry,* 1966, *122,* 841–851.

Langner, T. S. A twenty-two item screening score of psychiatric symptoms indicating impairment. *Journal of Health and Human Behavior,* 1962, *3,* 269–276.

Leighton, A. H., Lambo, T. A., Hughes, C. C., Leighton, D. C., Murphy, J. M., & Macklin, D. B. *Psychiatric Disorder among the Yoruba.* Ithaca, N.Y.: Cornell University Press, 1963.

Leighton, D. C., Harding, J. S., Macklin, D. B., Macmillan, A. M., & Leighton, A. H. *The Character of Danger,* New York: Basic Books, 1963.

Lemkau, P. *Mental Hygiene in Public Health.* New York: McGraw-Hill Book Company, 1949.

Lemkau, P., Tietze, C., & Cooper, M. Mental hygiene problems in an urban district. *Mental Hygiene,* 1942, *26,* 100–119.

Lipman, R. S., Rickels, K., Covi, L., Derogatis, L. R., & Uhlenhuth, E. H. Factors of symptom distress. *Archives of General Psychiatry,* 1969, *21,* 328–338.

Llewellyn-Thomas, E. The prevalence of psychiatric symptoms within an island fishing village. *Canadian Medical Association Journal,* 1960, *83,* 197–204.

Manis, J. G., Brawer, M. J., Hunt, C. L., & Kercher, L. C. Estimating the prevalence of mental illness. *American Sociological Review,* 1964, *29,* 84–89.

Markush, R., & Favero, R. Epidemiologic assessment of stressful life events, depressed mood, and psychophysiological symptoms—A preliminary report. In B. P. Dohrenwend & B.

S. Dohrenwend, (Eds.), *Stressful life-events: Their nature and effects.* New York: Wiley, 1974.

Martin, F. M., Brotherston, J. H. F., & Chave, S. P. W. Incidence of neurosis in a new housing estate. *Brit. J. Prev. Soc. Med.*, 1957, *11*, 196–202.

Meile, R., & Haese, P. Social status, status incongruence and symptoms of stress. *Journal of Health and Social Behavior*, 1969, *10*, 237–244.

Pasamanick, B., Roberts, D. W., Lemkau, P. W., & Krueger, D. B. A survey of mental disease in an urban population: prevalence by race and income. In B. Pasamanick (Ed.), *Epidemiology of Mental Disorder.* Washington, D.C.: American Association for the Advancement of Science, 1959. Pp. 183–191.

Paykel, E. S., Myers, J. K., Lindenthal, J. J., & Tanner, J. Suicidal feelings in the general population: A prevalence study. *British Journal of Psychiatry*, 1974, *124*, 460–469.

Pearlin, L. Sex roles and depression. In N. Datan & L. Ginsberg (Eds.), *Life-span developmental psychology: Normative life crises.* New York: Academic Press, 1975.

Pearlin, L., & Johnson, J. Marital status, life-strains and depression. Unpublished manuscript, 1975.

Phillips, Derek. 1966. "Rejection of the Mentally Ill: The Influence of Behavior and Sex." *American Sociological Review* 29 (October): 679–87.

Phillips, D. The "true prevalence" of mental illness in a New England state. *Community Mental Health Journal*, 1966, *2*, 35–40.

Phillips, D., & Segal, B. Sexual status and psychiatric symptoms. *American Sociological Review*, 1969, *34*, 58–72.

Primrose, E. J. R. *Psychological Illness: a Community Study.* London: Tavistock Publications, 1962.

Public Health Service. 1970. *Selected Symptoms of Psychological Distress.* Public Health Service Publication no. 1000, ser. 11, no. 37. Washington, D.C.: Government Printing Office.

Radloff, L. Sex differences in depression: The effects of occupation and marital status. *Sex Roles*, 1975, *1*(3), 249–265.

Rosanoff, A. J. Survey of mental disorders in Nassau County, New York, July-October 1916. *Psychiatric Bulletin*, 1917, *2*, 109–231.

Roth, W. F., & Luton, F. B. The mental hygiene program in Tennessee. *American Journal of Psychiatry*, 1943, *99*, 662–675.

Schwab, J. J., Brown, J. M., & Holzer, C. E. Sex and age differences in depression in medical inpatients. *Mental Hygiene*, 1968, *52*, 627–630.

Schwab, J. J., McGinnis, N. H., & Warheit, G. J. Social psychiatric impairment: Racial comparisons. *American Journal of Psychiatry*, 1973, *130*(2), 183–187.

Sethi, B. B. Personal communication to M. M. Weissman and G. W. Klerman. Lucknow, India, 1974.

Siassi, I., Crocetti, G., & Spiro, H. R. Loneliness and dissatisfaction in a blue collar population. *Archives of General Psychiatry*, 1974, *30*, 261–265.

Sorenson, A., & Stromgren, E. Frequency of depressive states within geographically delimited population groups. *Acta. Psychiat. Scand. Suppl.*, 1961, *162*(37), 62–68.

Srole, L., Langner, T. S., Michael, S. T., Opler, M. K., & Rennie, T. A. C. *Mental Health in the Metropolis.* New York: McGraw-Hill, 1962.

Strotzka, H., Leitner, I., Czerwenka-Wenstetten, G., & Graupe, S. R. Social-psychiatrische Feldstudie über eine ländliche Allgemeinpraxis. *Social Psychiatry* 1966, *1*, 83–87.

Tauss, W. 1967. "A Note on the Prevalence of Mental Disturbance." *Australian Journal of Psychology* 19 (August): 121–23.

Taylor, Lord, and Sidney Chave. 1964. *Mental Health and Environment.* London: Longman's Green.

Tsuwaga, T., Okada, K., Hanasiro, S., Asai, T., Takuma, R., Morimura, S., & Tsuboi, F. Uber die psychiatrische Zensusuntersuchung in einem Stadtbezirk von Tokyo. *Psychiatria et Neurologia Japonica*, 1942, *46*, 204–218.

Uchimara, Y., Akimoto, H., Kan, O., Abe, Y., Takahashi, K., Inose, T., Shimazaki, T., & Ogawa, N. Über die vergleichend psychiatrische und erbpathologische Untersuchung auf einer Japanischen Insel. *Psychiatria et Neurologia Japonica*, 1940, *44*, 745–782.

Weeke, A., Bille, M., Videbeck, T., Dupont, A., & Juel-Nielsen, N. Incidence of depressive syndromes in a Danish county. *Acta. Psychiat. Scand.*, 1975, *51*, 28–41.

Weissman, M. M., & Klerman G. L. Sex differences and the epidemiology of depression. *Archives of General Psychiatry*, 1977, *34*, 98–111.

Chapter 4

DEPRESSIONS AMONG WOMEN: THEIR NATURE AND CAUSES

Gerald L. Klerman
Myrna M. Weissman

INTRODUCTION

Previous chapters in this volume have examined in some detail utilization data from mental health facilities and have reviewed epidemiological data on mental health problems. Given these utilization data, it is clear that women are *not* overrepresented in mental hospital patient populations. It is clear, however, that women exceed men in their rate of treatment for depression. Moreover, there is considerable evidence from community surveys that untreated depression is disproportionately more prevalent among women (Weissman & Klerman, 1977). Furthermore, there is evidence that the rate of untreated depression, especially among young women, may be rising (Weissman, 1975).

A repeated conclusion in epidemiologic studies of depression is that women predominate. Observations of a sex difference in the frequency of any disorder attract attention and stimulate explanations. Depression has recently gained the attention of biologists, sociologists, feminists, and the educated public. Is it a true finding that women are more prone to depression? Or are the observations the result of confounding factors in case reporting or in the organization of the health care system? If the finding is "real," what processes, biological or psychosocial, best explain the differences?

The topic is timely for a number of reasons. All aspects of women's roles and experience are currently under scrutiny. Demographic changes in this century have increased longevity for women more than for men.

ISBN 0-12-310850-0

However, while these changes have resulted in a larger population of women aged 60–80, the greater number of older women in itself cannot account for the predominance of depressed women found in epidemiologic studies. The preponderance of women is not only in the absolute numbers of depressed patients, but, more significantly, in rates per population group adjusted for age. At every age group, rates of depression are higher for women. Moreover, there is evidence for a lowering in the modal age of onset of depression. Whereas pre-World War II textbooks characterized the age of onset of depression as the fourth decade of life, recent reports emphasize onset of depression in young adults, again females predominating.

A number of explanations for this showing have been offered. One set of explanations questions whether the finds are real and speculates that they are an artifact accounted for by women's perceptions of stress and by their coping responses, their willingness to express psychological symptoms, and the high rate at which they seek medical help. Alternatively, the finding is considered a true phenomenon and attributed to female biological susceptibility or to psychosocial causes.

How can these important sex differences be understood? To understand these trends, it is necessary to re-examine the nature of depression and its causes, and then analyze the causal explanations offered for the higher rates of depression among women. In this chapter, we will first review the most important current views on clinical depressions, their antecedents, and their consequences.

THE NATURE OF DEPRESSIONS

Descriptions of depressions are as old as written documents; recognizable accounts of depressive states occur in ancient Egyptian, Greek, and Biblical texts. Excellent portraits of depressed persons occur in Shakespeare's plays and in the novels of the eighteenth and nineteenth centuries.

Since the early part of this century, mental health clinicians and investigators have grouped the depressions and other related emotional states into the category of "affective disorders." Although a broad spectrum of symptoms, behaviors, and states are included within this category, the dominant feature common to these otherwise diverse disorders is that the patients' disturbance is expressed in their mood and emotional distress. As the most common conditions included among the affective disorders, the depressions are clinical states in which persistent abnormal emotional symptoms are associated with feelings of worthlessness, guilt, helplessness, and hopelessness; anxiety, crying, suicidal tendencies; loss of interest in work and other activities; impaired capacity to perform everyday social functions; and hypochondriasis, or bodily alterations including anorexia, weight change, and constipation; psychomotor retardation; and agitation.

Mania and other elations are the less frequently seen, but the more dramatic, conditions within the category of affective disorders. Most manic patients (over 80%) also have depressive episodes at some points in their lives, but the converse is not true: Only a small fraction of depressed patients (about 10%) also have manic episodes. However, the close association of these two affective conditions led Kraepelin and other nineteenth-century clinicians to define the manic-depressive illness category. While manic-depressive is one important form of depression, it represents only a small fraction of depressions and affective disorders.

Some authorities also include anxiety and tension in the affective disorders, but current research evidence supports the classification of anxiety states separately from depression. However, over one-half of depressed persons also experience anxiety, tension, and related symptoms.

Depressions are similar in many aspects to other broadly defined clinical syndromes in general medicine, like anemia, congestive heart failure, or jaundice. Like these other medical conditions, patients present common clinical features that may be due to diverse causes. The clinical depressive syndrome has the common feature of intensity of emotion and multiple etiological forces (genetic, environmental, or biochemical); it allows for multiple treatments such as psychotherapy, drugs, and so on.

Epidemiological studies in the United Kingdom, Scandinavia, and the United States have documented the fact that large proportions of individuals among the general population, and perhaps as many as 20–30% of all females experience depressive episodes at some point in their adult lives, often of moderate severity. However, only one-quarter of those with depressive symptoms and behaviors seek professional attention from physicians, let alone from psychiatrists. There is a large group of distressed individuals who, because of stigma, shame, or inability or unwillingness to gain access to medical care do not receive treatment.

The heterogeneity of the clinical manifestations within the depressive disorders should be emphasized. Though clinicians identify these depressed states on symptomatic and behavioral criteria, they would ideally like to make diagnoses based on etiologic criteria. This ideal is far from being realized in psychiatry in general, and in the affective disorders in particular. Multiple etiological factors are involved: genetic, biochemical, personality, stress and life events, and social background. Some affective syndromes, like the bipolar form of manic–depressive illness; (i.e. persons who have both highs and lows) almost certainly have major genetic determinants. Other depressions are the consequence of drugs such as amphetamines or rauwolfia. However, in the majority of depressions, the proximate etiology is uncertain and clinicians' and patients' explanations invoke varying combinations of stress, personality, changes in the central nervous system (CNS) catecholamines, and other factors. However, our current knowledge of these etiological factors is limited, and at best, relies on evidence far removed from the immediate clinical situation.

Some Problems of Terminology

The meaning of the term "depression" does not remain constant in different fields—neurophysiology, pharmacology, psychology, and psychiatry all employ the term, but with varying definitions. The resulting confusion makes some attempt at clarification of its psychiatric meaning and use appropriate. For the neurophysiologist, depression refers to any decrease in electrophysiological activity, as, for example "cortical depression." To the pharmacologist, depression refers to drug actions which decrease the activity of the target organ; thus the "CNS depressants" include the barbiturates and the anesthetics, which are not related clinically or pharmacologically to antidepressant drugs. The experimental psychologist uses the term "depression" for any decrement in optimal performance, such as a slowing of psychomotor activity or a reduction of intellectual functioning. For the clinical psychiatrist or psychologist, however, depression covers a wide range of changes in affective state, ranging in severity from the normal mood fluctuations of everyday life to severe melancholic psychotic episodes.

Unfortunately, the use of the same term in a number of scientific fields has perpetuated the view, and also the hope, that there are common mechanisms unifying the neurophysiological, pharmacological, and clinical phenomena. In the past, clinical psychopathological states have been ordered on a continuum according to alteration in patients' psychomotor activity; thus manic excitements were presumably due to excessive CNS excitation and were contrasted with depressive symptoms presumably due to inhibition of generalized or specific CNS functioning. This polarity concept has also been applied to Pavlovian conditioning and to psychoanalytic theory. Moreover, the selection of therapy was rationalized by this polarity model. Using the traditional classification of drugs into stimulant and depressant categories, treatment drugs were chosen if their actions were opposite to the presumed CNS activity. This "stimulant-depressant continuum" has been the classical model for drug treatment, and was popular during the period when the amphetamines and barbiturates were the major CNS agents. And recent proposals relating catecholamines to affective disorders parallel to the older characterization of a stimulant-depressant continuum. However, the complexity of actions of newer psychotropic drugs, particularly the phenothiazines and tricyclic depressants, makes the stimulant-depressant continuum model overly simplistic and obsolete. Lithium's actions in preventing recurrence of both manic and depressed episodes suggest that there are neurochemical processes common to both elation and depression or to one's predisposition to these states. In the absence of firmly established neurophysiological, biochemical, or even psychodynamic mechanisms in the etiology or pathophysiology of depressive disorders, assessment, diagnosis, and therapeutic decisions continue to be based almost entirely on clinical criteria.

Distinguishing Normal Mood from Depressive Illness

As a mood, depression is part of normal human living. The capacity to experience depression is part of humanity's evolutionary heritage and has contributed greatly to the survival and growth of the species. Feelings of sadness, disappointment, and frustration are within the vicissitudes of the human condition. The distinction between normal mood and abnormal depression is not always clear, and psychiatrists do not always agree on the full range of emotional phenomena to be diagnosed as pathological.

The fact that the depressions involve an accentuation in intensity and/or duration of otherwise normal emotions has mixed consequences for clinical judgment. On the one hand, this fact promotes the empathic understanding of clinicians and family members to patients' difficulties. Almost all human beings experience unhappy, sad, depressed, and discouraged periods, and thus it is often easy to identify the individuals' emotional state and empathize with his or her distress. However, this very familiarity sometimes renders clinical assessment and differential diagnosis difficult, in that there may be a lack of appreciation that the individual has crossed the boundary area between the normal and abnormal. Particularly among family and friends of the patients, there is a tendency to minimize the severity of the patient's difficulties because the manifestations may seem like a normal emotional state. Similarly, clinicians also tend to minimize the severity of affective reactions even when precipitating stressful events are apparent.

In severe forms, most depressed states are easily judged as pathological by criteria of intensity, pervasiveness, persistence, and interference with usual social and bodily functioning. The difficult problems arise in distinguishing normal states from the many mild depressive illnesses.

In addition to the dominant disturbances of mood, depressive illness usually involves some combination of the following features:

1. Impairments of bodily functioning, as manifested by disturbances in sleep, appetite, sexual interest, autonomic nervous system, and gastrointestinal activity.

2. Reduced desire and ability to perform usual expected social roles in the family, at work, in marriage, in school, etc.

3. Suicidal thoughts or acts.

4. Disturbances in perception, cognition, and reality testing, as manifested by delusions, hallucinations, confusion, etc.

While suicidal thought and acts and impairment of reality testing are relatively infrequent, their presence usually indicates that the patient's behavior is no longer to be considered in the range of normal mood swings, but requires psychiatric attention. Features indicative of depression are listed in Table 4.1.

The Depressive Syndromes

Very rarely do depressed patients experience only one of the many symptoms described; most often patients report multiple symptoms. The patient with a depressive illness usually manifests depressed mood plus a significant number (four to five) of other associated symptoms. Because

TABLE 4.1
Symptoms and Behaviors of States of Depressions

1. Depressed mood characterized by reports of feeling sad, low, blue, despondent, hopeless, gloomy, etc.
2. Changes in posture, facial expressions, speech, dress, grooming
3. Change in appetite, usually leading to weight loss
4. Sleep difficulty, usually insomnia
5. Loss of energy; fatigue, lethargy, anergy
6. Anxiety
7. Bodily complaints
8. Agitation (increased motor activity experienced as restlessness)
9. Retardation of speech, thought, and movements
10. Decrease in capacity to experience pleasure
11. Decrease in sexual interest and activity
12. Loss of interest in work and usual activities
13. Diminished ability to think or concentrate, with complaints or "slowed thinking" or "mixed-up thoughts"
14. Feelings of worthlessness, self-reproach, guilt, shame
15. Fall in self-esteem
16. Feelings of helplessness
17. Pessimism and helplessness
18. Thoughts of death and/or suicide attempts

some symptoms occur together with greater-than-chance expectation, terms such as "symptom configuration", "cluster", "constellation", or "syndrome" are used to refer to the coexistence and covariance of associated depressive symptoms and behaviors. Recently, factor analysis and other multivariate correlational statistics have been applied to symptom ratings and personality tests to identify such symptom groupings.

Moreover, it is important to recognize that there is no *one* depressive syndrome. There is no universal agreement as to the bases upon which the various depressive syndromes should be identified and separated. Most theorists and investigators accept the principle that heterogeneity exists within the affective disorders. The official nomenclature designates multiple affective states such as manic–depressive illness, involutional states, psychoneurotic depression, and so on. The retarded–agitated typology and the psychotic–neurotic separations are two conventional subtypes of depression which have been partially useful in clinical work. Other subtypes involve the primary–secondary separation and the endogenous–neurotic distinction.

THEORIES OF THE CAUSES OF DEPRESSIONS

Having described the characteristics of depressions as clinical states and some of the features that may distinguish the forms of it which should be treated from the normal mood, we will now review the major theories explaining this common condition currently under investigation. It should be noted that these theories usually refer to the problem of depression in general and not to the special problem of explaining the preponderance of this emotional condition among women. We shall address this latter issue in the next section of this chapter, after reviewing the general theories of depression.

Theories about depression have had a long and controversial history. Depressive syndromes have been ascribed to biological factors, social causes, stress reaction, and recently, to social labeling. The concept of depression as a mental illness, developed by Kraepelin during the late nineteenth century, has had, and continues to have, the greatest influence in the medical and psychiatric professions. His work on manic-depressive illness (Kraepelin, 1921) emphasized biological causation, mostly genetic and metabolic in nature, and allowed little room for social, environmental, or psychological explanations.

Adolph Meyer's (1957) theory of psychobiology offered an alternative to the nineteenth century conception of mental illness as exclusively biologically caused. Kraepelin's (1921) biological disease concept of depression and Meyer's reactive concept of depression continued to be theoretically opposed to each other for over 70 years. In 1933, Aubry Lewis (1967) offered evidence strongly contradictory to Gillespie's view of endogenous depression, and supporting Meyer's concept of depression as a psychobiological reactive form. In Western Europe and North America, most theorizing and teaching adopted Meyer's ideas of psychobiology and a unitary view of depression. This unitary view of depression emphasized the common features among various types of depressive episodes, and stressed the continuity between every day "moods," mild depression, and psychotic episodes of melancholia. According to this theory the vicissitudes of the life experience were a possible cause of depression. The Meyerian perspective tended to minimize classification systems, and to downplay the importance of constitutional and genetic factors.

Currently, theorists and clinicians tend to hold that neither Kraepelin's concept of depression as a disease, nor the Meyerian view of depression as a reaction form, is completely satisfactory. But definitional confusion and disagreement about terminology has seriously hampered the progress of research on depression. Recently, there has been an upsurge of interest in biological theories, emphasizing hereditary, hormonal, and genetic influences in the incidence of depression. Since World War II, treatment has concentrated on psychotherapeutic methods. The host of highly effective antidepressant drugs developed over recent years have focused discussion and research on the interaction between biological and psychosocial explanations of depression.

Loss and Stress

The most widely held theory about depression relates its onset and quality to the stress accompanying loss and separation. This theory is based upon the close similarities between the normal emotional reactions to loss and separation and the clinical state of depression. The prototype of the reaction to loss and separation is, of course, that of grief and mourning which follows the death of a loved one. The emotional, behavioral, and biological similarities of the grief and mourning state to clinical depression have been observed for centuries, and since the beginning of modern psychiatry, have formed the basis for psychological understanding of the state. There is good anthropological and comparative animal behavioral data indicating that the capacity to become depressed is based upon the evolutionary heritage of the human species, in reactions to loss, and that the response of humans is similar to that of animals. The responses of children to loss and separation have been widely studied, particularly by psychoanalysts such as Spitz (1946), A. Freud (1965), and Bowlby (1969).

It is their observations that have formed the basis for the loss theory. Similarly, observations of reactions of adults to catastrophe and disaster, such as those made by Lindemann (1944) in the Coconut Grove fire disaster, indicate that the grief and mourning state may, if not adequately resolved, lead to clinical depression as well as to other clinical states.

In recent years, the concept of loss has been extended to include not only separation and death, but also symbolic losses and other forms of threats to self-esteem and impairment of interpersonal relations. This extension has generated a considerable amount of clinical and theoretical controversy.

The concept of loss has also been broadened to include the general concept of stress, particularly after the studies of Selye (1956) on the hormonal and physiological responses of organisms to various forms of stress. Research efforts to quantify stress using the techniques of Holmes and Rahe have led to fruitful research which indicates that among depressed patients, experiences of loss and separation occur more frequently than they do in a matched normal sample. However, direct loss and separation cannot account for all forms of depression; thus it is necessary to include in the concept of loss symbolic loss and other forms of stress.

Psychodynamic Theories

The literature concerning the psychodynamic variables involved in depression in extensive. It also becomes increasingly complex as qualifications are added to the earliest Freudian theories to account for evidence from personality and sociological research. However, most psychodynamically oriented workers agree that the depressive condition is related to personality needs, especially orality, internalized aggression, strong superego, and extreme narcissism. Furthermore, they hypothesize that the early years of life are especially important in forming the individual's predisposition to adult depression. Theorists often disagree as to the role of superego factors in depression and the intrapsychic mechanisms and identifications found in depression. Freud (1957), Abraham (1927), and the classic psychoanalysts depicted depression as a basically hostile response to a lost love object. The hostility, in the process of being repressed, is turned against the self, and clinically results in self-destructive impulses. The neo-Freudians have directed attention to interpersonal functioning as part of the broadening of psychodynamic thinking and clinical experience. Widely held views about the predisposing personalities of depressives emphasizes that depression-prone people are inordinately dependent on others in order to maintain their own self-esteem. Their frustration tolerance is low and they employ a variety of techniques such as manipulation, submission, coercion, pity, and demands to maintain those desperately needed but still ambivalent relationships with external or internalized objects (Bonime, 1976).

These ideas have had extensive influence on theory and clinical practice. They are most influential in psychotherapeutic practice. But extensive research efforts have only partially verfied their scientific bases (Chodoff, 1972, 1974), and until further evidence is generated, the psychodynamic theories must be regarded as stimulating but still tentative and not fully established.

Genetic Transmission Theories

Extensive evidence supports the existence of a genetic factor causing or predisposing certain individuals toward depression. Family studies have examined the rates of illness within families, and the evidence indicates that affective disorders are more likely to occur in first degree relatives of diagnosed patients than in the general population (Klerman & Barrett, 1973). Twin studies which compare illness rates for monozygotic twins indicate that they show a higher concordance rate for affective disorders. Crossrearing studies following high-risk children raised in adoptive homes (Kety, Rosenthal, Wender, Schulsinger, & Jacobson, 1975) attempt to separate out the proportional influence of genetics and environment. These types of family studies indicate a genetic basis for at least an inherent vulnerability to depression, particularly the manic–depressive forms.

A more sophisticated method for studying the genetics of depression is linkage studies, in which known genetic markers are used to follow traits throughout the family network. X-linkage markers are particularly important for testing sex differences in rates of depression disorder. If the gene for depression is located in the X chromosome and the trait is dominant, females, who have two X chromosomes, will be more often affected than males, who have only one X chromosome. However, if the trait is recessive, males will be more often affected than females. However, different types of depression, such as in bipolars and unipolars, complicate the testing of the X-linkage hypothesis. Some family studies demonstrate X-linkage transmission for unipolars, but not for bipolars, while others suggest the opposite; still others provide no evidence at all for any sex linkage.

Kidd, Reich, and Kessler (1974) proposed a polygenic model of inheritance in addition to the conventional single genic pattern. Perhaps there exists a genetically determined differential threshold to stress in the environment, with women having a lower threshold and therefore greater susceptibility to a depressive response to specific environmental stresses.

Pharmacological and Neurochemical Theories

Drug-related research in the last 10 years has produced an intriguing neurochemical theory of depression. This line of research has generated the amine hypothesis of affective disorders, which relates depression to a functional deficit of one of more brain neurotransmitter amines at specific central synapses. Conversely, mania, in this view, is associated with a functional excess of one or more or these amines. There are critical synapses in brain areas which are related to vegetative and affect regulatory behavior. Norepinephrine, dopamine, and serotonin are the neurotransmitter amines regulating the flow of impulses in these brain areas. At the synaptic junction, the neurotransmitter serves as a chemical transducer which converts electrical energy into chemical energy, which is then reconverted into electrical energy. Complex processes are responsible for synthesis, storage, release, re-uptake, and metabolism of the amine neurotransmitters. When electrical impulses arrive at the nerve endings, the storage granules containing norepinephrine release some of the transmitter substance, which then reacts with the receptor and causes an electrochemical event at the receptor site.

Two concurrent pharmacological observations initiated the amine hypothesis. The first occurred in the treatment of hypertension with reserpine, when it was observed that a large proportion of patients so treated for hypertension became depressed (Goodwin & Bunney, 1971). Another research team (Shore & Brodie, 1957) finds that reserpine depleted serotonin and norepinephrine in the brain. Monoamine oxidase (MAO) inhibitor drugs are capable of elevating brain amine levels, and in animals, treatment with MAO inhibitors could inhibit or reverse symptoms of depression caused by reserpine.

Another piece of evidence appeared with the tricyclic antidepressants. Although they do not directly alter the amine levels in the brain, they do block the presynaptic re-uptake of the amines so that there is a functional increase in amines at the synaptic juncture. Lithium, an effective drug in the treatment of mania, enchances the re-uptake of amines at the synapse, therefore lowering the amount of amines at the synaptic cleft. These drug actions indirectly support the general hypothesis that depression is a deficit of brain neurotransmitter amines and that mania is an excess of these amines at specific synapses.

This amine theory, in the ensuing years, required modification according to the different classifications of depression (i.e., unipolar and bipolar) and mania, and the pharmacological responses to the many types of drugs by those taking them. Unexpected reactions of patients responding or not responding to certain drug therapies in opposition to what was anticipated suggest that the chemical interactions and shifts during depression are extremely complex, and that more careful research is necessary.

Cognitive Theories

Many clinicians and researchers have hypothesized that the psychological deficit in depression involves a cognitive problem. Beck (1974) in particular has studied the cognitive themes of depressed patients. These patients misinterpret or exaggerate the real or imagined loss, and attach extravagant meanings to their difficulties. The depressed person views everything in his life, his attributes, his relationships, and his achievements with a sense of inadequacy and failure, past, present, and future. In his sufferings, the depressed person attributes the cause of the difficulty to himself. A chain reaction is triggered in which the patient personalizes the defect, magnifies any deficiencies, devastates his own self-esteem, and then harshly reproaches and criticizes himself. Pessimism alternates with apathy as the patient regards his own state of affairs. In dreams and in verbal productions, depressed patients center on three interdependent themes: a negative view of the self, of the outside world, and of the future. Beck suggests that this set of idiosyncratic patterns, which he labels the "cognitive triad," pervades the conscious experiences of the depressed person.

One strength of this cognitive model lies in its potential for a new psychotherapy. An extremely low self-concept can be treated by presenting a hierarchy of cognitive tasks and to demonstrate, through these tasks, the invalidity of the patient's self-reproaches. This allows the therapist not only to generally approve of the depressed person, but to offer an objective evaluation of the patient's ability to perform a cognitive task.

Attempts have been made to specify what types of reinforcement for a cognitive task are more likely to raise self-esteem. Dweck (1975) hypothesizes that a person who has learned helplessness believes failure to be a result of his absence of ability or a result of external factors beyond his control. A person who believes failure to be a result of his own lack of motivation will be likely to escalate his effort in an attempt to obtain a goal. The cognitive theory, a relatively recent one, attempts to link experimental psychological research with clinical observation and systematic therapeutic intervention.

Behavioral Approaches

Behavior theory views depression in stimulus and response terms. Depression is characterized by a reduction in the frequency of many kinds of activity and an increase in the frequency of others, usually avoidance and escape. The depressed person's complaints, requests, bizarre behaviors, and repetitions are, functionally speaking, avoidance and escape behaviors, since they are reinforced by the removal of the aversive stimulus. Moreover, there is a deficit of positively reinforced activities in a depressed person's repertoire. The psychological treatment often consists of restoring the normal balance between negatively and positively reinforced activities.

Ferster (1974) identifies some specific behavior mechanisms that account for the frequency of the depressed person's actions and thus explain, in part, the infrequency of certain activities by the depressed person. He hypothesizes that fixed reinforcement schedules which require a large and regular amount of activity for each reinforcement are more apt to produce depression than variable reinforcement schedules. For instance, he suggests that the housewife and the professional who are both performing within a standard routine are more susceptible to depression than the struggling young executive or substitute teacher in a school system. According to Ferster, the uncertainty and variability in the reinforcement for the young executive and substitute teacher are less likely to produce strain than the stiff schedule associated with a stable work situation in which a constant daily amount of activity is needed to achieve a required goal.

Changes in the person's environment, or within himself, produce a disorientation and a shifting of dependable reinforcers. When changes are too drastic, the person may not be able to locate reinforcers for his particular repertoire of behaviors, and so may choose not to act. This lack of acceptable positive reinforcers, it is theorized, produces depression.

A low frequency of positively reinforced behaviors perpetuates the distorted perception of the patient's own inability to influence the environment. Low frequency of verbal activity indicates a patient's unwillingness to interact with the environment and to locate specific negative and positive contingencies in the environment. In Ferster's words (1974), "The patient has (1) a limited view of the world, (2) a 'lousy' view of the world, and (3) an unchanging view of the world [p. 39]."

Lewinsohn (1974) used this social reinforcement model as the basis for his behavioral approaches. He observes that a low rate of response-contingent, positive reinforcement elicits certain aspects of the depressive syndrome, such as inactivity, fatigue, etc. The low rate of response-contingent, positive reinforcement is predicted by three factors: potentially reinforcing events in the environment, the availability of reinforcement in the environment, and the instrumental behavior of the individual. Depression is predicted when there is little probability that the individual's behavior will be followed by positive reinforcement and when there is great probability that the individual will be reinforced when he does not emit the behavior. Depressed persons are observed to be deficient in social skills; that is, they lack the ability to behave in such a way as to receive positive reinforcement from others. Measures of social skill, such as amount of behavior, modes of interaction, interpersonal range, positive reactions, and action latency indicate the patient's lack of interest in either giving or receiving positive reinforcement in their social interactions.

Learned Helplessness Theories

Recent experiments on animal behavior have created a condition in animals that parallels depression in humans. Seligman (1975) observes that dogs, after receiving a few trials of inescapable shock, accepted shock passively, without attempting to escape. The dog "learned" that it could not control the shock, and that no response succeeded in producing relief; the dog thus "learned" that it was totally "helpless." Continued laboratory trials suggested that an animal which had "learned helplessness" had extreme difficulty in "learning" that there were times when a response would produce relief from shock.

The behaviors of learned helplessness in animals are similar to features of clinical depression. One outstanding similarity is passivity. Animals and humans who have experienced an inability to control reinforcing contingencies in their environment thereafter demonstrate fewer voluntary responses, acting less on their own initiative. Helpless animals and depressed people also maintain a negative, cognitive set. That is, they have difficulty learning that their own responses can produce useful outcomes. The pessimism of the depressed patient is focused on his own inability to act in a skillful and influential enough manner to produce a change or reaction to anything or anyone in his surroundings. A third similarity between learned helplessness and depression relates to the timing of depression. If helplessness is induced in animals by a single session of uncontrollable shock, that sense of helplessness will dissipate in time. But if the animal undergoes multiple trials of inescapable shock, the helplessness persists for longer periods. In humans, a single catastrophic incident, such as the death of a child, produces grief and a sense of depression. This form of extreme depression is usually relieved with the passage of time. But if a person is subjected to continued experiences of inability to control what is happening in his life, there is a likelihood that he will maintain the symptoms of a depression for a longer time. The fourth similarity, that of lessened aggression, is the subject of much controversy in the field of depression. Helpless animals initiate fewer aggressive and competitive responses, and their status within the group diminishes. In the same way, clinically depressed patients seldom act in an aggressive or hostile manner, although the content of their dreams and conversation may be intensely aggressive. Helpless animals and depressed humans act alike in that they both will manifest loss of appetite, loss of weight, and lack of interest in sexual behavior. There are also strong similarities in the physiological and chemical changes that accompany the behaviors, although the chemical basis of depression has not been completely explicated. Helpless rats show norepinephrine depletion, while antidepressant drugs have the common ability to increase norepinephrine available at certain brain synapses.

In addition to these similarities, Seligman (1975) argues that helplessness is caused by learning that responding is independent of reinforcement; or in depression terms, that action is futile. Contrary to many other theories of depression, Seligman's holds that it is not the loss of reinforcement, but the loss of *control* over reinforcement that causes depression.

Relating Behavioral and Biological Theories

Seligman's theory of learned helplessness in animal studies and depression in humans has been challenged by physiological evidence. Laboratory experiments (Weiss, Glazer, & Pohorecky, 1974) indicate that the animal's inability to effectively act in the learned helplessness situation is due to a decrease of the norepinephrine in the animal's brain. The neurochemical shift is caused by environmental stress; when the stress, such as inescapable shock, is relieved, the neurochemical levels slowly return to normal, and the helpless animal then regains the ability to respond instrumentally.

Evidence that there is this biochemical mechanism rather than a learning mechanism derives from a series of animal studies. Helpless dogs, when tested 24 hours after inescapable shock, fail to jump the hurdle, but dogs tested 48 hours after inescapable shock can and do respond by jumping. This suggests that the early lack of response was due not to a learning phenomenon, but rather to a temporary biochemical depletion. Supplementary experiments with rats make this hypothesis more tenable. A group of rats exposed to a $3\frac{1}{2}$ minute swim in cold water which reduced brain norepinephrine levels could not respond to avoid shock immediately afterwards. However, animals swimming in warm water showed no difficulty in escaping shock. But since norepinephrine primarily affects motor activity, rats in warm or cold water were shown to be able to avoid shock by responding to a task which required little motor activity, such as poking their noses through a hole to shut off the shock. In addition, drugs which are known to compensate for decreased norepinephrine levels protect animals against response deficits in a learned helplessness paradigm.

This biochemical–behavioral research is intriguing because it relates stress to brain norepinephrine levels. It offers a possible mechanism for relating the chemical theories of depression to behavioral theories of depression, and accommodates both the catecholamine hypothesis of norepinephrine depletion in the brain and the environmental theories that implicate stress as a causative factor in clinical depression. However, there are still too many gaps in the research to allow for any conclusive synthesis of the findings.

It is apparent that there is no final agreement as to the causes of depression. Although there is moderate agreement among clinicians as to the differences between clinical states and the normal emotional mood of depression, this concordance does not extend to the causes of the depressive syndromes, not to the best manner as to the classification of the various clinical states. Increasingly, it is being recognized that a single cause is unlikely to emerge, and that more complex, multicausal explanations are necessary to understand this complex human experience.

EXPLANATIONS FOR PREPONDERANCE OF WOMEN SUFFERING FROM DEPRESSION[1]

There is very good evidence that rates of depression amongst the sexes differ, both in the United States and elsewhere. Various explanations have been offered for this sex difference. There is a possibility that the trends are spurious, caused by faults and inconsistencies in the varying methods of reporting symptoms. The sex differences may be real and attributable to the biological susceptibility of women due to genetic factors or to the female endocrine system; or to psychosocial factors such as social discrimination; or to the learned helplessness of women.

Evidence that Women Predominate among Depressives

The available evidence of the predominance of females among depressives comes from four sources: observations of patients coming into treatment; community surveys of persons not under treatment; studies of suicide and suicide attempters; and studies of grief and bereavement. These data are reviewed in earlier chapters of this book and in Weissman and Klerman (1977).

Some of the sex variations in depression rates can be explained by differences in methodology, particularly in case definition. However, the methodological difficulties notwithstanding, it is striking that the findings show, with amazing consistency, a preponderance of females among depressives.

Of the various sources of evidence, the most compelling are from community surveys. Since rates of treated cases do not represent true

[1] The material in this section of the chapter derives in large part from abstracting Weissman, M. M., and Klerman, G. L. Sex differences and the epidemiology of depression, *Archives of General Psychiatry*, 1977, *34*:98–111.

prevalence, epidemiologic analysis requires data from community surveys. Such surveys usually involve a random sample drawn from a total community, and therefore provide information on many persons who have the disorder but have not received treatment.

Data are available from a number of community surveys in the United States and elsewhere. In clinical studies of diagnosed cases, the sex ratios show some minor variations; but in the community surveys, there are no variations, with the exception of bereaved widows, who will be discussed separately. Women predominate in all countries and all time periods.

The Problem of Artifact Due to Reporting of Stress and Symptoms

There have been frequent discussions as to whether this predominance of women among those diagnosed as depressed may be an artifact of the methodology. Reports from data sources as diverse as clinical observations, community surveys, and suicide studies indicate that women are overrepresented in the diagnostic category of depression. Are women really more depressed, or do they show up in the statistics more often for other reasons? Perhaps this preponderance of women is the result of their more frequently being under stress; perhaps to their willingness to admit to stress. Or maybe women's response biases make them appear to be more depressed. It is possible that the same stress has different effects on men and women. Variations in the help-seeking patterns of men and women may mean that more female depressives show up in doctor's offices and therefore represent a larger proportion of the statistics.

Are Women under More Stress?

Before the sex differences in rates of depression can be regarded as an artifact, the possibility must be considered that women are under more stressful life events and therefore run a greater risk of succumbing to depression. Many clinicians, observing that stressful events occur before the onset of clinical depression, concluded that these events precipite the depression. Holmes and Rahe (1967) provided great impetus to these studies by developing a simple quantitative scale for assessing the life events used in epidemiologic and clinical studies. Their results support the hypothesized relationship between stressful life events and the onset and severity of numerous medical illnesses and psychiatric disorders, particularly depression. Consistent sex differences in stress reports have appeared.

Uhlenhuth, Lipman, Balter, and Stern (1974) conducted elegant studies to examine the relationship between actual and perceived stress, using newer life events scales and reports of symptoms by patients in both psychiatric settings and normal populations in community studies. Uhlenhuth *et al.* find a direct relationship between stress and symptom intensity, but do not find that women reported more stressful life events. At the same levels of stress, women reported symptom intensities about 25% higher than men. This study was repeated with similar results in a probability sample of all households in Oakland, California.

Dohrenwend (1973) and others discuss the thesis that life event stresses act in an additive manner with health problems of all kinds. The basic hypothesis is that stressful life events include all major life changes, whether positive or negative. Most life event scales measure stresses as dramatic as divorce or loss of spouse, loss of job, relocation, and also minor stresses, like giving up smoking or changing a typical routine. Major life event stresses are equally distributed between men and women. However, it is possible that the minor stresses associated particularly with the role of married women may have been previously underweighted in the scoring of life event scales, and should be given much more importance in assessing a woman's susceptibility to depression. New life event scales (Atkinson, 1975) are being developed and tested to more accurately depict the subtle and relative stresses on men and on women.

Current stress scales emphasize discrete life events and acute changes in life conditions. They are relatively insensitive to certain chronic conditions such as poverty, large family size, or health problems, which might have a greater impact on women than men. However, pending empirical research, the available evidence is that women do not experience or report more stressful events.

Do Women Weigh Events as More Stressful?

While women may not report experiencing greater numbers of stressful life events, they may evaluate these events as more stressful than do men. To study the weight given to stress, Paykel, Prusoff, and Uhlenhuth (1971) asked patients and their relatives to judge the degree to which various life events were upsetting. They found no sex differences. Men did not appear to evaluate the standard lists of life events as having a very different impact upon their lives than did women.

Women Report More Symptoms, Especially of Affective Distress

One hypothesis proposed to account for the excess of depressive symptoms among women is that women respond to stress with affective distress because they feel freer to acknowledge symptoms. Clancy and Gove

(1974), examining the possible role of social disapproval in the reporting of symptoms and find no significant sex difference. Women did not report more desire for social approval than men did; neither did they judge having psychiatric symptoms as less undesirable than did men. Clancy and Gove conclude that sex differences in symptom reporting appear to reflect actual differences and are not an artifact of response bias: women actually experienced more symptoms.

Women Go to Doctors More Often

Women cope with problems by visiting doctors, and, by every measure of utilization of the general health care system, women predominate. They have higher rates than men of use of outpatient facilities, of visiting physicians, of getting prescriptions, and taking psychotropic drugs.

Consistent with this are the findings for seeking help. Women will come for aid for minor complaints. Women seek treatment for depression more often, while men have a higher suicide rate. In our society, the public assumption of the role of being sick is interpreted by men as a sign of weakness. Moreover, the health care system is organized in ways that make it difficult for most men to get treatment, since office hours usually conflict with hours of employment. But help-seeking patterns alone cannot account for the predominance of depressed women in community surveys, since the majority of persons classified as depressed in community surveys have not been treated in psychiatric clinics, and thus have not been included in any official treatment rates.

Alcoholism and Deviance

The male-female statistics are more balanced if one considers alcoholism as a disorder and compares rates of alcoholism among men and women with those for depression. Apparently families and social conventions can tolerate depressed women and alcoholic men, but not depressed men and alcoholic women (Winokur, Rimmer, & Reich, 1971). Perhaps depressed men drink in order to lessen their feelings of despair physiologically (Mayfield, 1968) or emotionally, through their drinking groups. Alcoholic patients often have serious depressive symptoms (Tyndel, 1974); clinically depressed patients often have histories of alcoholism (Reich, Davies, & Himmelhoch, 1974). Although studies have solidly linked alcoholism and depression, the causal sequence is still unclear.

However, the two types of behavioral deviance, that is, depression and alcoholism, lead to very different directions of help seeking. While women predominate in the health care system, men predominate as inmates in correctional institutions. Better reporting by traditional psychiatric facilities and correctional institutions could more accurately depict the role of depression in the institutionalization of men and women.

More males than females have alcohol problems; thus some unknown proportion of depressed men appear in the alcoholism rates but are not identified as depressed. There are debates, however, as to whether or not these men are really depressed. Accurate diagnostic assessments are required to determine the morbid risk of depression and the time of its onset in relation to the beginning of the alcoholism problem. Similar factors must be considered regarding the possibility that depressed men are to be found in the correctional system. Pending future research, this remains an interesting, but unproven, hypothesis.

When all these possibilities are assessed, our conclusion is that the female preponderance is not an artifact.

The Female Preponaerance Is Real and Is Possibly Due to Biological Factors

We conclude that the sex differences are real findings and now must examine the possible explanations. Some of the hypotheses involve biological susceptibility; among these, the investigations have been made as to the role of genetic transmission and of female endocrine physiological processes.

The possibility that there is a genetic factor in the etiology of depression has regularly attracted attention. There are four main sources of evidence for the genetic hypothesis: family aggregation studies, which compare illness rates within and between generations of a particular family based on the fact that members of the same family share the same genes to varying degrees; studies of illness rates in monozygotic and dyzygotic twins; cross-rearing studies; and linkage studies, in which known genetic markers are used to follow other traits through several generations or in siblings. The majority of genetic research in depression is concerned with evidence from family aggregation or twin studies.

The available evidence summarized by several investigators shows an increased morbid risk of affective disorder in the first-degree relatives of diagnosed patients as compared with the general population, and a higher concordance rate for affective disorders in monozygotic than dyzygotic twins. Taking into consideration all the studies, there is reasonable evidence of the existence of a genetic factor operating in depression.

Much of the recent evidence suggests X-linkage for inheritance of the manic–depressive form of depression. This mode of genetic transmission could explain unequal female–male rates. However, the available evidence is limited in quantity and inconsistent in direction, and pending further research, the genetic explanation must be acknowledged as possible, but not established.

Interest in the possible relationships between female sex hormones and affective states derives from observations that clinical depression tends to occur in association with events in the reproductive cycle, including the menstrual cycle, the use of contraceptive drugs, the postpartum period, and menopause. The female endocrine system has been widely proposed as the cause of mood swings and affective disorders in women. Yet many women accept premenstrual tension, postpartum depression, and menopausal changes as expected realities in their lives.

Ivey and Bardwick (1968) report that anxiety (measured by analyses of verbal samples) peaks during the premenstrual phase. Thirty to 50% of the 839 women responding to the Moos Menstrual Distress Questionnaire (Moos, 1968, 1969) reported that cramps, backache, headache, irritability, mood swings, and/or depression were associated with menstruation. Coppen and Kessel (1963) find through their questionnaire that premenstrual symptoms are significantly correlated with neuroticism. Zimmerman and Parlee (1973), who analyze cyclic phase and its relation to mood swings, find no significant differences between phases.

However, recent critical reviews, such as Sommer (1973) and Parlee (1972), describe the methodological problems inherent in many of these hormonal studies that may distort results. Other inaccuracies may arise from individual variations in the cycle phase among women examined and by response biases among the women surveyed. Many women often describe themselves as being tense, irritable, anxious, and depressed about 4 to 5 days before the onset of menses (see Moos, 1968, 1969, Paige, 1971). Parlee (1973) administered the Moos Menstrual Distress Questionnaire to both male and female subjects with instructions that they should "describe symptoms that women sometimes experience" during the menstrual and premenstrual phases of the cycle. Both women and men selected similar types of symptoms in response to Parlee's questioning. Although a number of physiological and psychological theories have been offered to explain the premenstrual syndrome, none of them convincingly presents a coherent biological process as the cause of estrogen drop and mood changes. There is still not sufficient evidence to conclusively link depression with the menstrual cycle.

However, the postpartum period is one phase of the life cycle where research provides solid data implicating hormones in mood changes. The significant hormonal shifts after giving birth are accompanied by mood disturbances. In the postpartum period, women do have a higher rate of serious psychiatric disorders, especially depression. Several studies which surveyed admission rates in psychiatric facilities (Paffenbarger & McCabe, 1966, Pugh, Jerath, Schmidt, & Reed, 1963) verified the increase in psychoses and mental disorders during the first to third month after delivery.

A concurrent finding is that pregnant women are *less* likely to be incapacitated by mental disorders (Gordon & Gordon, 1959). Researchers can not yet define how specific endocrines and endocrine changes influence postpartum psychiatric illness and protect against prenatal mental illness. It is clear that the social and emotional factors surrounding the birth of a child may contribute to this pattern as much as the concurrent hormone levels do.

The menopausal period of a woman's life is often depicted as a particularly depressing time. This has historically and officially been labelled involutional melancholia. Symptoms such as agitation, hot flushes, obsessions, and hypochondriasis increase. Depression has commonly been believed to accompany this change in life. But in an extensive study of over 800 women aged 38–60 (Hallstrom, 1973), no significant differences in the one-year incident rates of mental illness or depressive states were found in the different age categories. And Winokur (1973b) finds that there is no greater risk of depression during menopause than during other times of the life span. Thus a category of menopausal depression causally related to regular hormonal activity is not currently tenable.

The pattern of the relationship of the female endocrine system to clinical states is inconsistent. There is good evidence that premenstrual tension and use of oral contraceptives increase depressive mood, but these effects are probably of small magnitude. There is excellent data to show an increase in depression in the postpartum period. Contrary to widely held views, there is good evidence that the menopause does not increase rates of depression.

But there is little to substantiate a finding relating these mood changes and clinical states to altered endocrine balance or specific hormones. No study could be located which correlated clinical state with female endocrines, utilizing modern endocrinological methods or sensitive quantitative hormonal assays. Here is an area for fruitful collaboration of further research between endocrinology and psychiatry. As of now, it can be said that while some portion of the sex differences in depression, probably during the childrearing years, may be explained endocrinologically, this factor is not sufficient to account for the large ratio of sex differences in rates of depression.

Psychosocial Explanations

Psychologists, sociologists, feminists, and others concerned with women's problems have increasingly looked to psychosocial factors to explain why more women than men become depressed. The conventional wisdom holds that the longstanding disadvantaged social status of women has psychological consequences that result in depression. This persistence of social status discrimination is proposed to explain the long-term trends of female predominance in depression. In addition to this hypothesis, explanations based on views of female personality and on historical changes associated with social stress are offered.

Psychological Disadvantages of Women's Social Status

Various hypotheses have been proposed specifying the ways in which women's disadvantaged status might contribute to their pronounced rates of clinical depression. Our review of these hypotheses indicates two main pathways. One emphasizes the low social status, and the legal and economic discrimination against women; the other focuses on women's internalization of role expectations, which results in a state of learned helplessness.

The first pathway, which we call the *social status hypothesis,* is widely accepted in the recent discussions of social discrimination against women. Many women find their life situations depressing, since real social discriminations make if difficult for them to achieve mastery by direct action and self-assertion, which only further contributes to their psychological distress. It is suggested that these inequities lead to legal and economic helplessness, dependency on others, chronically low self-esteem, low aspirations, and ultimately, clinical depression.

The second pathway, which we call the *learned helplessness hypothesis,* proposes that socially conditioned, stereotypical images produce in women a cognitive set against assertion, which is reinforced by societal expectations. In this hypothesis, the classic "femininity" values are redefined as a variant of the "learned helplessness," characteristic of depression. Young girls learn to be helpless during their socialization and thus develop a limited response repertoire when under stress. These self-images and expectations are internalized in childhood so that the young girl comes to believe in the stereotype of femininity, especially its emphasis on youthfulness, beauty, and passivity.

Women and Learned Helplessness

The findings of the learned helplessness experiments of Seligman (1974, 1975) have been extrapolated to apply to the social status of women. Although the learned helplessness theory does not provide any immediate explanations for the sex difference in depression, certain aspects of the theory are particularly apt in describing the situation of women. Women are particularly susceptible to loss because they generally depend more than men upon social statuses, which are easily lost. Today's greater geographic and economic mobility mean that women are more likely to leave family and friends as they move and establish themselves in new jobs and in new neighborhoods. Within the family, the man's dependence on a job takes priority over the woman's dependence on her socioemotional network. Therefore women realistically may have less of a sense of control over their lives, and greater feelings of helplessness and loss.

As for treatment, if we look at animal experiments, the most effective way to overcome learned helplessness in dogs is to force them to respond. In other words, dogs must be *made* to jump in order to avoid shock. For the depressed patients, there are many therapies geared to teach the patient that she or he can solve a problem or perform a task. Electroconvulsive shock has also been shown to be effective in reducing depression and helplessness in humans and dogs. The prevention of succumbing to learned helplessness depends on the person's previous experience in mastering reinforcements in his or her own behavior. In depression, people who have been victimized, with few opportunities to influence positively and change their uncomfortable situation, are particularly susceptible to depression.

The role of women throughout history and even currently in our society is marked by a sense of powerlessness, an inability to produce a substantial influence on the course of events. The stereotypical feminine role tends to be defined as passive. The stereotypical areas of expertise for females, such as housework and cooking, tend to become not so much a matter of mastery as of routine.

Women's roles and occupations are seldom evaluated honestly. Therefore, it is thought, women, because of their roles, are predisposed to feelings of learned helplessness over a considerable period of time. If, because of their less powerful social roles, women have experiences which reinforce their feelings, of helplessness, they are likely to acquire depressive symptoms. This correspondence between Seligman's concepts of learned helplessness and the powerlessness of women's roles in society has been explicated more clearly and carefully by various feminist theorists.

Marital Role and Depression

In one of the few attempts to test the hypothesis that the high rates of depression are related to the disadvantages of women's social status, particular attention has been given to the difference in rates of mental illness of married and unmarried women. If the social status theory is correct, marriage should be a greater disadvantage to the woman than to the man, since married women are then more likely to fulfill the traditional stereotyped role and should, therefore, have higher rates of depression. Gove (1972), in particular, has researched rates of mental illness among married women as compared to the rate among unmarried women and married men.

Studies about the role performance of depressed women provide information about social conflicts of depressed patients. In a matched study, Weissman, Klerman, Paykel, Prusoff and Hanson (1974) observed that depressed women are extremely impaired in their roles as spouse, mother, and participant in close family relationships. Relationships with friends and extended family relations cause less difficulty for the depressed women. It appears that depressed women who are employed outside the home exhibit fewer differences in social functioning than comparable nondepressed women. Depressed women, then, are less maladjusted in instrumental roles than in expressive roles.

Based on these findings, Mostow and Newberry (1975) studied women workers and housewives coming for treatment of depression. In the initial sample, there appeared to be no significant difference in the severity and type of depression experienced by 21 matched worker and housewife subjects. After 1 month of treatment, the mental states of the two groups of sample subjects were still similar to each other. However, after 3 months, there were indications that the worker women were beginning to adjust socially while the housewives reported impaired performance, disinterest, feelings of inadequacy, and economic difficulties. It is important to consider that the working women were participating in sterotypically nongratifying jobs, such as those falling in the 4 and 5 categories of the Hollingshead Scale, and yet they still felt more competent than the housewives at their work. This is an indication that the work role, at any level, can support and benefit the depressed woman.

The association of poor interpersonal relations within the marriage and clinical depression is further supported by studies of depressed women during psychiatric treatment. The New Haven group (Paykel *et al.*, 1969) finds that marital discord was the most common event reported by depressed patients as having occurred in the previous six months. Weissman and Paykel (1974) found that acutely depressed women as compared to matched normal groups reported considerably more problems in marital intimacy, especially in their ability to communicate with their spouses. Moreover, these marital problems often were enduring and did not completely subside with symptomatic remission of the acute depression.

The strains of the marriage role were cited by Gove (1972) as a causal factor in higher rates of mental illness among women. Since the selective process of marrying filters out the mentally ill, the married of both sexes have lower rates of mental illness than the unmarried. However, Gove (1972) indicates that an important sex difference occurs in the rates of mental illness among married persons. Being married "protects" men against mental illness; for women, however, marriage produces difficulties which promote mental illness. The married woman's role is usually more stressful since it involves only one major source of gratification, the home life. The role of housewife is unstructured and invisible, with self-imposed rather than objective standards of performance. Also, many of the women's instrumental roles, such as the jobs they often fill, are frustrating, involve little skills and few challenges, and are not very prestigious. If a married woman does work outside the home, she is generally in a less satisfactory position in terms of pay, upward mobility, and scheduling. The expectations for a woman are unclear and diffuse. Rather than attaining clearcut individual goals, women spend much time adjusting to external contingencies.

On the other hand, the roles of single men and women are fairly similar, particularly for jobholders lacking close interpersonal ties. But after marriage and/or divorce, rates of depression among women are higher than among men, suggesting that women must cope with more role conflicts outside their control than men.

The data showing that unmarried women have lower rates of mental illness than unmarried men, but that married women have higher rates than married men, are cited as evidence that the excess of symptoms in married women is not entirely due to biological factors intrinsic to being female, is partly caused by the conflicts generated by the traditional female role.

Psychoanalytic Explanations

Among mental health clinicians, a widely held explanation for the high rates of depression among women attributes it to women's specific intrapsychic conflicts. Interestingly, two relatively independent psychoanalytic theories related to this issue developed in the early decades of this century, but theories were not linked together until recently with the emergence of the feminist critique. One is the psychoanalytic theory of female psychological development; the other, psychodynamic theory of the psychogenesis of depression.

As to the former, Freud and other psychoanalysts proposed that the personality of adult women, normal and neurotic, is characterized by narcissism, masochism, low self-esteem, dependency, and inhibited hostility, as a consequence of the young girl's special resolution of her Oedipal complex. This theory had been extensively criticized by Clara Thompson and Karen Horney, and more recently by Kate Millett. The classic psychodynamic theory of depression emphasized that individuals prone to depression had difficulties in close relationships, showed excess dependency, had suffered early childhood deprivation, felt excessive guilt, and manifested a tendency to turn hostility against themselves. According to this theory, the immediate precipitant for the overt clinical depression was hypothesized to be a loss, either actual or symbolic.

These two theories grew parallel with each other for almost 50 years. But few psychoanalysts attempted to link the epidemiologic fact that women predominate among depressives with their presumed characteristic psychic conflicts regarding narcissism, low self-esteem, dependency, and childhood experiences of penis envy. Although these two theories have been widely accepted among clinicians in one form or another, empirical evidence to support them has been meager.

The Possible Contribution of the Mental Health System

The prominence of these psychodynamic views among clinicians has stimulated criticism of the mental health system by feminists. They claim that women's difficulty in freeing themselves from the feminine stereotype has been consistently reinforced in public by "experts" on child development and psychology. Keller, Kirsh and other critics assert that psychotherapeutic treatment too often reiterates the negative self-image of women and perpetuates problems of women suffering symptoms arising from their life situations.

The most often-quoted work on the existence of sex role stereotypes among mental health professionals was undertaken by Broverman, Broverman, Clarkson, Rosenkrantz, and Vogel (1970), who asked mental health clinicians what behaviors they considered healthy in men, women, and adults whose sex was unspecified. The study found a powerful negative assessment of women. The standard for a healthy adult was the same as that for a healthy man but *not* as for a healthy woman. Healthy women were seen as differing from healthy men in that the healthy women were supposed to be submissive, dependent, subjective, emotional, and easily hurt. Thus, a double standard of mental health was found which parallels the sex-role stereotypes in our society. Moreover, both sexes incorporated the best or worst aspects of the stereotypical role in their image of themselves; women tended to have a more negative self-image than men.

Feminist critics have been intense in their assertions that psychiatry is a male-oriented profession which has perpetuated male-dominated theories (Chester, 1972). Attempts have been made to encourage women to seek female therapists and to join groups for consciousness-raising. Before these feminist criticisms can be accepted, the results of studies on the attitudes and views of female mental health practitioners need to be appraised. From these studies, it can be seen that, in response to various case histories, male psychotherapists judged protocols of female patients less stringently than did female counselors. Thus, male mental health professionals were not necessarily bound by their ideology to discriminate against women.

How well psychiatric theory can explain depression in women has been strongly debated in recent years. Some believe that psychoanalytic theory does not provide a coherent personality system for women, nor the model of a strong, nonstereotypical woman. A number of critics (Franks & Burtle, 1974) assert that the mental health practice continues to support stereotyped roles for women by concentrating on women in relationship to their love objects—men—as fathers or spouses. They say that psychotherapy places a woman in a passive stance as a patient, encouraging expressiveness and a transference of trust to the psychoanalyst.

This is a crucial attack since the majority of therapists and psychiatrists who work with women are men. Case studies and experimental studies have pointed up sex discrimination and sexual preoccupation in therapy (Masling & Harris, 1969). Observations of testing sessions have indicated that male mental health professionals extended treatment sessions for females and used more sexual romantic projective tests and discussions with women (Barocas & Vance, 1974).

This suspicion of the male mental health professional has encouraged the use of female therapists and psychiatrists. Feminist therapists have organized and proclaimed themselves as more able to understand and deal with the mental health needs of women. However, some recent studies (Abramowitz & Abramowitz, 1973) indicate that female mental health practitioners are, in fact, quicker to infer greater maladjustments in females than in males. There is as yet little evidence to suggest that males support sex stereotypes in their depressed female patients more so than do female professionals. It appears that mental health personnel of both sexes maintain stereotypical and sex-biased notions or role adjustments.

Labeling Theory and Professional Stereotypes

Building on these findings, labeling theorists would explain the sex differences in depression not as an artifact in methodology or help-seeking patterns, but rather as a consequence of professional behavior. These theorists cite society's reaction to and labeling of symptoms as the source of any differences in diagnoses patterns. Szasz (1970), for instance, holds that a diagnosis of mental illness tends to produce conformity to society's standards (Szasz, 1970). Scheff's (1966) influential sociological approach proposes that virtually everyone at some time commits an act that corresponds to the public stereotype of mental illness. If and when the public acknowledges these acts, the person, depending on his status in society, may be labeled as mentally ill. These views place the onus of diagnosis on external standards and evaluations in mental health.

A major factor in the labeling of mental illness is the sex of the individual patient. The Broverman *et al.* (1970) study of clinicians' evaluations of mental health documented the existence of sex-role stereotypes among mental health professionals. The existence of such stereotypes has led to speculation that the diagnosis of depression is a labeling category applied selectively to women. The sex differences in rates of depression, according to this view, are "caused" by the labeling process, rather than to the actual differences in the numbers of men and women suffering from depression.

Although it is clear that professional and societal attitudes towards sex roles influence the diagnosis and treatment of depression, the labeling view seems too simplistic to explain the complicated interaction between sex role and depression. For example, it cannot explain why in epidemiological studies, women consistently describe themselves as much more depressed than men. In epidemiological studies, societal labeling and stereotyping are not influencing factors. However, both the stereotypic female role and women's attitudes toward themselves within that role may contribute to the higher likelihood of women to maintain the symptoms of and be diagnosed with depression. Yet this does not seem to be the explanation for the high rates of women among untreated depression cases.

Historical Change, Rising Expectations, and Increasing Rates of Depression among Women

Any attempt to understand the female preponderance in depression must explain both the long-term and the short-term trends. Conventional explanations have assumed that the female predominance in depression has been a long-term trend. Data from the nineteenth century does indicate a female predominance of depression. That these trends are longstanding can be interpreted as supporting either the biological or the social status theory.

On the other hand, recent evidence suggests short-term trends. There has been an increase in the rates of depression, especially among young women, manifested by their rising rate of suicide attempts and by the high attendance of women at psychiatric outpatient clinics. This has prompted speculation about the possible contributory role of recent social changes, especially the presumed increased psychological stresses of modern life.

Rising expectations, changing demographic trends, increased life events, separations, and loss of attachment bonds are all factors creating risks of depression which have been suggested as mechanisms by which social change can create psychic stress. It is proposed that these stress factors have a greater impact on women because of their more vulnerable social position.

Increases in depression have been reported during other periods of rapid social change. The possible historical parallels to the current era in the late Elizabethan and early seventeenth century England, when depression was described to have reached epidemic proportions, have been described. One explanation during this period attributed the rise in mental illness to the "wear and tear of a civilization," and speculated on the reasons for the sex differences in rates of prevalence of mental disorder.

Rising expectations, access to new opportunities and efforts to redress the social inequalities of women have been suggested as possible explanations for the recent increase in depression among women. Depressions may occur not when things are at their worst but when there is possibility of improvement, and a discrepancy between one's rising aspirations and the likelihood of fulfilling these wishes. The women's movement, governmental legislation, and efforts to improve educational and employment opportunities for women have created higher expectations. But social and economic achievement often have not kept pace with the promises, especially in a decreasing job market, where long-standing discriminatory practices perpetuate unequal job opportunities.

These new role expectations may also create personal conflicts, particularly for women who value their traditional family tasks but who also desire employment and recognition outside the family. While the women's movement has mainly involved middle- and upper-class and educated women, it has had an impact on women from other social classes where opportunities for work outside the home, management of money, and dominance in the marriage may be crucial. Even for the educated and economically comfortable women, ambivalence and conflict continue about careers not conventionally seen as feminine. The documented increase in suicides and suicide attempts among women suggests that social changes may be exacting psychological costs for many young women. In this regard, Gove and Tudor (1973) note that communities which are extremely closeknit, stable, traditionally family-oriented, and culturally isolated, have lower rates of mental illness in general, with the women having even lower rates than the men.

Although support can be adduced for the hypothesis that participation in the women's movement is associated with psychological distress, it is unlikely that this is a major factor for the high rate of depression among women. The rate differences long predate the women's movement. While short-term changes may be disruptive, over a long period, a new equilibrium may be reached and the high female rates may begin to decrease. Such a reduction in women's rate of depression would be indirect confirmation of the hypothesis that the excess of depression among women is due to the psychological disadvantages of the female role. As social behaviors of the sexes become more equivalent, females may begin to employ modes of coping with stress similar to those used by men. There are some indications that the female rates of alcoholism, suicide, and crime—which are usually male behaviors—have begun to rise. Alternatively, the sex ratios for depression could become equal because of an increase in depression among men due to the stress produced by the new status of women, and the uncertainty of the male role. In this regard, it would be interesting to determine the rates of depression among educated and emancipated women. Similarly, are the rates of depression equalized between the sexes in cultural subgroups where sex role allocations are less rigid or nonconventional?

Summary of the Psychosocial Explanations

The most convincing evidence that social role plays an important role in the vulnerability of women to depression is the data that suggest that marriage has a protective effect for males but a detrimental effect for women. This supports the view that elements of the traditional female role may contribute to depression. Further understanding of social stress and its interactions with components of female vulnerability in the traditional role is a promising area of research. This research would need to take into account intervening variables such as women's employment and the quality of their marriages. Any comprehensive theory, including those based in biological explanations, must account for both the long-term rates and recent changes in rates.

CONCLUSIONS

The male–female differences in rates of depression are real. The evidence in support of these differential rates is best established in Western industrialized societies. Further studies in non-Western countries, particularly in Africa and in Asia, are necessary before any conclusions can be drawn as to the universality of these rate differences.

There is little doubt, however, that the sex differences found in depression are a promising lead which require a considerably broader based inquiry in epidemiology. It is highly unlikely that any one of the explanations already described will account for the phenomena, nor that every type of depressions will be associated with the same risk factors. As was shown, the explanations cross such a wide variety of disciplines that it is rare to find one group of investigators entertaining all of them. There has been an unfortunate tendency for fragmentation, so that the investigators in genetics, social psychology, or endocrinology are not specifically aware of attempts by colleagues in other fields to deal with similar phenomena. The purpose of this review has been to assess different positions and, hopefully, to guide future research.

We propose an integrative theory based on the concept of adaptation. Clinical depression is a maladaptive outcome of partially successful attempts of adaptation (Klerman, 1974). To support this thesis, Klerman has reviewed the adaptive functions of emotions and affects, especially sadness and depression, throughout the evolutionary process: social communication, physiological arousal, subjective awareness, and psychodynamic defense. Evidence for the communication function of affects came from the separation–loss paradigm in animal studies (Harlow, Harlow & Suomi, 1971). A baby monkey separated from the biological mother, cloth mother, or peers communicates the need for maternal or peer support with actions that replicate the affect of depression. Just as separated animals maintain a fear–flight–arousal system, the depressed human is preparing for meeting and dealing with dangers. A "conservation-withdrawal" response, as seen by Schmale and Engel (1967), involves reduced activity, lowered metabolism, and increased parasympathetic activity.

Internalized and subjective affects also play important functions in psychic reflection. They permit goal-setting and self-evaluation, which are again representative of evolutionary attainments. Psychodynamic thinking has stressed the important role of affect in stimulating defense mechanisms which protect against danger to the ego's self-esteem. It is clear from these examples that the affective state of depression has been adaptive, from an evolutionary perspective, particularly for primates and human infants.

The adult depressive, however, still utilizes patterns such as dependency, passivity and helplessness, which were once adaptive in the child's developmental schemes, but are useless in the adult. The depressive episode is often initiated as a response to helplessness and fallen self-esteem, but this attempted adaptation fails. Depression does not facilitate social communication and interpersonal relationships. It does not prepare the organism to meet with the environmental contingencies. It causes a misperception in awareness of self, and employs defensive mechanisms that have negative consequences.

A combined model of learned helplessness and life event stresses with concurrent physiological changes may accommodate a new theory about the development of depression which accounts for the sex differences found in depressive symptoms. According to the sociopsychological explanation for depression, we could expect to find the highest rates of depression among that group of people who experience the greatest number of stressful events life demands, and at the same time the fewest actual possibilities for mastery of them.

We suggest that a balance of external stress and individual vulnerability predisposes women to this maladaptive response. While stress does contribute to the timing and precipitation of acute depressive episodes, stressful events are not universal or specific to depression. We advocate an adaptive model to integrate external stress and internal physiological and psychological balances. We foresee a future theory that will accommodate and link loss and separation changes, social order, genetic vulnerability and changes in the CNS biogenic amines. Animal studies testing the various effects of antidepressant drugs with concurrent behavioral indices will help to specify particular chemical-behavioral relationships. It is clear that different types of drug therapies, such as tricyclical antidepressants, monoamine inhibitors, estrogens, and so on, prove to have varying degrees of effectiveness on certain classifications of depression. All the evidence supports a pluralistic theory of the causes and treatments of depressions.

REFERENCES

Abraham, K. *Selected papers of Karl Abraham, M.D.* London: Hogarth Press, 1927.

Abramowitz, S. I., & Abramowitz, C. V. Should prospective women clients seek out women practitioners? Intimations of a "ding-bat" effect in clinical evaluation. *Proceedings, 81st Annual Convention, American Psychological Association*, 1973, *8*(1), 503–504.

Atkinson, C. Personal communication, 1975.

Barocas, R., & Vance, F. Physical appearance and personal adjustment counseling. *Journal of Counseling Psychiatrists*, 1974, *21*, 96–100.

Beck, A. T. The development of depression: A cognitive model. In Friedman, R. J., & Katz, M. M. (Eds.), *The psychology of depression: Contemporary theory and research.* Washington, D.C.: V. H. Winston and Sons, 1974.

Bonime, W. The psychodynamics of neurotic depression. *Journal of the American Academy of Psychoanalysis*, 1976, *4*, 301.

Bowlby, J. *Attachment.* New York: Basic Books, 1969.

Broverman, I. K., Broverman, D. M., Clarkson, F. E., Rosenkrantz, P. S., & Vogel, S. R. Sex-role stereotypes and clinical judgments of mental health. *Journal of Consulting and Clinical Psychology*, 1970, *34*(1), 1–7.

Chesler, P. *Women and madness.* New York: Doubleday, 1972.

Chodoff, P. The depressive personality. Archives of General Psychiatry, 1972, *27*, 666.

Chodoff, P. The depressive personality: A critical review. In Friedman, R. J., & Katz, M. M. (Eds.), *The psychology of depression: Contemporary theory and research.* Washington, D.C.: V. H. Winston and sons, 1974.

Clancy, K., & Gove, W. Sex differences in mental illness: An analysis of response bias in self reports. *American Journal of Sociology*, 1974, *80*(1), 205–216.

Coppen, W. R., & Kessel, N. Menstruation and personality. *British Journal of Psychiatry*, 1963, *109*, 711–721.

Dohrenwend, B. S. Life events as stressors: A methodological inquiry. *Journal of Health and Social Behavior*, 1973, *14*, 167–175.

Dweck, C. S. The role of expectations and attributions in the alleviation of learned helplessness. *Journal of Personality and Social Psychology*, 1975, *31*(4): 674–685.

Ferster, C. B. Behavioral approaches to depression. In Friedman, R. J., & Katz, M. M. (Eds.), *The psychology of depression: Contemporary theory and research*. Washington, D.C.: V. H. Winston and Sons, 1974.

Fleiss, J. L. *Statistical methods for rates and proportions*. New York: Wiley, 1973.

Franks, V., & Burtle, V. (Eds.). *Women in therapy: New psychotherapies*. New York: Brunner/Mazel, 1974.

Freud, A. *Normality and Pathology in Childhood*. New York: International Universities Press, 1965.

Freud, S. Mourning and melancholia. In *Standard Edition of the Complete Psychological Works of Sigmund Freud*, Vol. 14. London: Hogarth Press, 1957.

Goodwin, F. K., & Bunney, W. E., Jr. Depression following reserpine: A reevaluation. *Seminars in Psychiatry*, 1971, *3*, 435.

Gordon, R., & Gordon, K. Social factors in the prediction and treatment of emotional disorders of pregnancy. *American Journal of Obstetrical Gynecology*, 1959, *77*, 1074–1083.

Gove, W. R. The relationship between sex roles, marital status, and mental illness. *Social Forces*, 1972, *51*(1), 34–44.

Gove, W., & Tudor, J. Adult sex roles and mental illness. *American Journal of Sociology*, 1973, *78*, 812–835.

Hallstrom, T. *Mental disorder and sexuality in the climacteric*. Goteberg, Sweden: Orstadius Boktrystreu A. B., 1973.

Harlow, H. F., Harlow, M. K., & Suomi, S. J. From thought to therapy: Lessons from a primate laboratory. *American Scientist*, 1971, *59*,538–549.

Holmes, T. H., & Rahe, R. H. The social readjustment rating scale. *Journal of Psychosomatic Research*, 1967, *11*, 213–218.

Ivey, M., & Bardwick, J. M. Patterns of affective fluctuation in the menstrual cycle. *Psychosomatic Medicine*, 1968, *30*, 336–345.

Kety, S. S., Rosenthal, D., Wender, P. H., Schulsinger, F., & Jacobsen, B. Mental illness in the biological and adoptive families of adopted individuals who have become schizophrenic: A preliminary report based on psychiatric interviews. In Fieve, R. R., Rosenthal, D & Brill, H. (Eds.), *Genetic Research in psychiatry*. Baltimore: Johns Hopkins University Press, 1975.

Kidd, K. K., Reich, T., & Kessler, S. Sex effect and single gene: The relevance of sex effect in discriminating between genetic hypotheses. In Weissman, and Klerman, unpublished manuscript, 1975.

Klerman, G. L. Depression and adaptation. In Friedman, R. J. & Katz, M. M. (Eds.), *The psychology of depression: Contemporary theory and research*.

Klerman, G. L., & Barrett, J. E. The affective disorders: Clinical and epidemiological aspects. In Gershon, S., & Shopsin, B (Eds.), *Lithium: Its role in psychiatric research and treatment*. New York: Plenum, 1973.

Kraepelin, E. *Manic-Depressive Insanity and Paranoia*. Edinburgh: E. and S. Livingstone, 1921.

Lewinsohn, P. M. "A Behavioral Approach to Depression." In Friedman, R. J., & Katz, M. M. (Eds.), *The psychology of depression: Contemporary theory and research*. Washington, D.C.: V. H. Winston and Sons, 1974.

Lewis, A. *Inquiries in Psychiatry*. New York: Science House, Inc., 1967.

Lindemann, E. The symptomatology and management of acute grief. *American Journal of Psychiatry*, 1944, *101*, 141.

Masling, J., & Harris, S. Sexual aspects of TAT administration. *Journal of Consulting Clinical Psychology*, 1969, *33*, 166–169.

Mayfield, D. G. Psychopharmacology of alcohol: I. affective change with intoxication, drinking, behavior and affective state. *Journal of Nervous Mental Disorders*, 1968, *146*(4), 314–321.

Meyer, A. *Psychobiology: A Science of Man*. Springfield, Ill.: Charles C Thomas, 1957.

Moos, R. H. The development of a menstrual distress questionnaire. *Psychosomatic Medicine*, 1968, *30*, 853–867.

Moos, R. H. Typology of menstrual cycle symptoms. *American Journal of Obstetrics and Gynecology*, 1969, *103*, 390–402.

Mostow, E., & Newberry, P. Work role and depression in women: A comparison of workers and housewives in treatment. *American Journal of Orthopsychiatry*, 1975, *45*(4), 538–548.

Paffenbarger, R., & McCabe, L. The effect of obstetric and prenatal events on risk of mental illness in women of child-bearing age. *American Journal of Public Health*, 1966, *56*, 400–407.

Paige, K. E. Effects of oral contraceptives on affective fluctuations associated with the menstrual cycle. *Psychosomatic Medicine*, 1971, *33*, 515–537.

Parlee, M. B. Comments on "roles of activation and inhibition in sex differences in cognitive abilities" by Broverman, Klaiber, Kobayashi, and Vogel. *Psychological Review*, 1972, *79*, 180–184.

Parlee, M. B. The premenstrual syndrome. *Psychological Bulletin* 1973, *80*(6), 454–465.

Paykel, E. S., Meyers, J. K., Dienelt, M. N., Klerman, G. L., Lindenthal, J. J., & Pepper, M. P. Life events and depression: A controlled study. *Archives of General Psychiatry*, 1969, *21*, 753–760.

Paykel, E. S., Prusoff, B., & Uhlenhuth, E. H. Scaling of life events. *Archives of General Psychiatry*, 1971, *25*, 340–347.

Pugh, T. F., Jerath, B. K., Schmidt, W. M., & Reed, R. B. Rates of mental disease related to childbearing. *The New England Journal of Medicine*, 1963, *268*(22), 1224–1228.

Reich, L. H., Davies, R. K., & Himmelhoch, J. M. Excessive alcohol use in manic-depressive illness. *American Journal of Psychiatry*, 1974, *131*(1), 83–86.

Scheff, T. *Being mentally ill: A sociological theory*. Chicago: Aldine, 1966.

Schmale, A. H., & Engel, G. L. The giving up-given up complex illustrated on film. *Journal of the American Psychoanalytic Association*, 1967, *15*, 344.

Seligman, M. E. P. Depression and learned helplessness. In Freedman, R. J. & Katz, M. M. (Eds.), *The psychology of depression: Contemporary theory and research*. Washington, D.C.: V. H. Winston and Sons, 1974.

Seligman, M. E. P. *Helplessness: On depression, development, and death*. San Francisco: W. H. Freeman, 1975.

Selye, H. The Stress of Life. New York: McGraw Hill, 1956.

Shore, P. A., & Brodie, B. B. Influence of various drugs on serotonin and norepinephrine in the brain. In Garattini, S. & Ghetti, V. (Eds.), *Psychotropic drugs*. Amsterdam; Elsevier, 1957).

Sommer, B. The effect of menstruation on cognitive and perceptual-motor behavior: A review. *Psychosomatic Medicine*, 1973, *35*(6), 515–534.

Spitz, R. A. *Anaclitic Depression: The Psychoanalytic Study of the Child*, vol. 2. New York: International Universities Press, 1946.

Szasz, T. S. Repudiation of the medical model. In Sahakian W. S. (Ed.), *Psychopathology Today*. Itasca, Ill.: F. E. Peacock, 1970.

Tyndel, M. Psychiatric study of one thousand alcoholic patients. *Canadian Psychiatric Association Journal*, 1974, *18*(1), 21–24.

Uhlenhuth, E. H., Lipman, R. S., Balter, M. B., & Stern, M. Symptom intensity and life stress in the city. *Archives of General Psychiatry*, 1974, *31*, 759–764.

Weiss, J. M., Glazer, H. I., & Pohorecky, L. A. Neurotransmitters and helplessness: A chemical bridge to depression? *Psychology Today*, 1974, 58–60.

Weissman, M. M. Depressed women: Traditional and nontraditional therapies. In *Effective psychotherapy*. Symposium presented at the meeting of the Texas Research Institute of Mental Sciences, Houston, November 1975.

Weissman, M. M., & Klerman, G. L. Sex differences and the epidemiology of depression. *Archives of General Psychiatry*, 1977, *34*, 98–111.

Weissman, M. M., Klerman, G. L., Paykel, E. S., Prusoff, B., & Hanson, B. Treatment effects on the social adjustment of depressed patients. *Archives of General Psychiatry*, 1974, 30(June), 771–778.

Weissman, M. M., & Paykel, E. S. *The depressed woman: A study of social relationships*. Chicago: University of Chicago Press, 1974.

Winokur, G. Depression in the menopause. *American Journal of Psychiatry*, 1973, *130*(1), 92–93.

Winokur, G., Rimmer, J., & Reich, T. Alcoholism IV: Is there more than one type of alcoholism? *British Journal of Psychiatry*, 1971, *118*, 525–531.

Zimmerman, E., & Parlee, M. B. Behavioral changes associates with the menstrual cycle: An experimental investigation. *Journal of Applied Social psychology*, 1973, *3*(4), 335–344.

Chapter 5

RISK FACTORS FOR DEPRESSION: WHAT DO WE LEARN FROM THEM?

Lenore Sawyer Radloff

The fact that depression is more common among woman than men has been thoroughly documented (see Chapters 3 and 4 of this book), but it is important to go beyond this basic epidemiologic finding and ask why. Empirically, this question translates first to asking under what conditions are women more depressed, and whether there are conditions under which women are *not* more depressed than men. These conditions can then be examined for underlying commonalities related to etiologic theories of depression. In other words, the research question changes from "Why are women more depressed than men?" to "What kinds of people are most likely to be depressed?" What do they have in common, and what does this tell us about the nature of depression?

DEFINITIONS OF DEPRESSION

Klerman and Weissman, in Chapter 4, have described the variety of definitions of depression and its symptoms. A diagnosis of clinical depression depends on the pattern of symptoms and on their severity and duration. One way of classifying the symptoms of unipolar depression is into a syndrome of four dimensions. The *cognitive dimension* includes hopeless, helpless beliefs—the conviction that nothing will ever get better. The irony of depression is that the person feels that nothing can help, whereas, in fact, depression can be quite effectively treated. The *motivational-behavioral dimension* includes feeling apathetic, lacking in energy,

ISBN 0-12-310850-0

not wanting to do anything, and actually doing less than usual. Depression often interferes with normal activities. It especially disrupts interpersonal relationships. The *affective dimension* includes feeling sad, blue, depressed, and taking no pleasure in the things that were formerly enjoyed. Depressed persons also often feel irritable and anxious, even quite openly angry and hostile, especially with the people closest to them (Weissman & Paykel, 1974). The trouble is that the anger is not used to communicate and to solve problems, but simply to express distress. It may be that the depressed person's low self-esteem and anger toward self comes from an awareness of his or her inadequate coping rather than from some mysterious turning of anger inward. The so-called *"vegetative" dimension* includes disturbances of appetite and sleep. Most commonly, depressed people have insomnia and do not feel like eating, but some sleep much more than usual, and overeat. These symptoms usually appear only in fairly severe depression (McLean, 1976).

There are many ways of measuring depression. In the data reported here, degree of depression will be operationally defined as the score on a depression scale, the Center for Epidemiologic Studies Depression Scale, referred to as the CES-D scale (see Table 5.1). The score consists of the number of symptoms of depression experienced during the past week, weighted by the frequency and duration of each symptom. A higher score indicates a higher level of depression. The scale includes many of the symptoms listed in Klerman and Weissman's Table 4.1 (Chapter 4) as characteristic of depression (for more information about the CES-D Scale, see Radloff 1977: and Weissman, Sholomskas, Pottenger, Prusoff, & Locke, 1977).

THE SURVEY DATA

The data presented in this chapter came from a mental health interview survey sponsored by the Center for Epidemiologic Studies, National Institute of Mental Health, conducted in Kansas City, Missouri in 1971–1972 and in Washington County, Maryland in 1971–1973. Individuals aged 18 years and over were randomly selected for interview from a representative sample of households. Response rates were 74.8% in Kansas City; 80.1% in Washington County.

The racial compositions of the samples reflected those of the populations. There were about 24% nonwhite in Kansas City, and only 2% nonwhite in Washington County. Preliminary analyses suggested that the whites and nonwhites should not be combined because they might differ in relationships among some variables. But the numbers of nonwhites were

TABLE 5.1
Center For Epidemiologic Studies Depression Scale (CES-D Scale)[a,b]

DURING THE PAST WEEK	RARELY	A LITTLE	MODERATE	MOST
1. I was bothered by things that usually don't bother me	0	1	2	3
2. I did not feel like eating; my appetite was poor	0	1	2	3
3. I felt that I could not shake off the blues even with help from my family or friends	0	1	2	3
4. I felt that I was just as good as other people	3	2	1	0
5. I had trouble keeping my mind on what I was doing	0	1	2	3
6. I felt depressed	0	1	2	3
7. I felt that everything I did was an effort	0	1	2	3
8. I felt hopeful about the future	3	2	1	0
9. I thought my life had been a failure	0	1	2	3
10. I felt fearful	0	1	2	3
11. My sleep was restless	0	1	2	3
12. I was happy	3	2	1	0
13. I talked less than usual	0	1	2	3
14. I felt lonely	0	1	2	3
15. People were unfriendly	0	1	2	3
16. I enjoyed life	3	2	1	0
17. I had crying spells	0	1	2	3
18. I felt sad	0	1	2	3
19. I felt that people disliked me	0	1	2	3
20. I could not get going	0	1	2	3

[a] Instructions for questions: Below is a list of the ways you might have felt or behaved. Please tell me how often you have felt this way during the past week (Hand card A): *Rarely* or none of the time (less than 1 day); some or a *Little* of the time (1–2 days); Occasionally or a *Moderate* amount of time (3–4 days); *Most* or all of the time (5–7 days).

[b] Total score equals the sum of the 20 weighted item scores.

too small to analyze separately in detail. Therefore, we shall cover analyses of whites only, with a sample size of 876 whites in Kansas City and 1639 whites in Washington County. Numbers in the various analyses will differ somewhat, due to missing data.

The survey operation was managed by local organizations[1] in each

[1] Fieldwork by Epidemiologic Field Station, Greater Kansas City Mental Health Foundation, Kansas City, Missouri; and Johns Hopkins Training Center for Public Health Research, Johns Hopkins University, Hagerstown, Maryland; under contract from Center for Epidemiologic Studies, National Institute of Mental Health.

site, and coordinated by the Center for Epidemiologic Studies to maintain the greatest possible comparability between the sites. Previous analyses of the data indicated that there was a small difference between the sites on the depression scale, but it disappeared when adjustments were made for racial composition and socioeconomic variables (Comstock & Helsing, 1976). Relationships among variables were very similar for the two sites. Therefore, the data from the two sites have been combined for the present report.

The questionnaire used in this survey included over 300 separate questions, including the CES-D Scale. The present analyses will cover only the CES-D Scale and some of the more objective sociodemographic factors which previously have been found to relate to depression (Silverman, 1968).

Overall, the average scores on the depression scale were higher for women than for men. However, this was true only among the married, the divorced–separated, and the never-married who were not heads of their own households (mostly young people living with parents). Among the widowed and the never-married heading their own households, the men's scores were higher than the women's. (see Table 5.2). (See also Radloff, in press and Radloff, 1975 for related analyses.)

Table 5.3 shows that other social factors associated with more depression for both sexes included youth (those of age 18–24 were more depressed than all other age groups), low education, low income, low status employment and physical illness (current or recent). Among males, but not females, currently employed workers were less depressed than others. For

TABLE 5.2
Average Depression Scores (CES-D), by Sex and Marital Status[a]

	MALE		FEMALE		TOTAL	
MARITAL STATUS	*N*	$\bar{x}$	*N*	$\bar{x}$	*N*	$\bar{x}$
Married	778	7.33	930	9.53	1708	8.53
Divorced–separated	66	7.89	145	13.71	211	11.89
Never-married (not head of household)	71	10.27	61	12.79	132	11.43
Never-married (head of household)	51	9.84	87	7.93	138	8.64
Widowed	45	12.78	267	10.26	312	10.62
Total	1011	7.94	1490	10.10	2501	9.23

Two-Way Analysis of Variance
Interaction sex × marital status $p = .0001$ (p values rounded)
Sex $p = .03$
Marital status $p = .0001$

[a] Higher score indicates more depressive symptomatology.

TABLE 5.3
Average Depression Scores (CES-D), by Sex and Other Social Factors

	MALE		FEMALE		TOTAL	
	N	$\bar{x}$	*N*	$\bar{x}$	*N*	$\bar{x}$
Age[a]						
18–24	146	10.51	189	13.48	335	12.19
25 & up	866	7.51	1296	9.62	2162	8.78
Education[a]						
Less than high school	375	8.27	608	11.22	983	10.09
High school	331	8.52	507	10.00	838	9.41
Beyond high school	304	6.94	369	8.44	673	7.76
Income[a]						
Less than $4000	121	10.06	311	11.58	432	11.16
$4000 or more	827	7.70	1034	9.47	1861	8.68
Occupational Status[a]						
High-level professional	45	5.76	5	2.80	50	5.46
Mid-level professional	100	6.11	69	8.14	169	6.94
Low-level professional	98	7.39	33	8.24	131	7.60
Sales & Clerical	88	7.50	181	8.73	269	8.33
Skilled manual	207	7.25	22	11.77	229	7.69
Semi-skilled manual	108	8.99	100	10.91	208	9.91
Unskilled manual	42	8.74	41	9.73	83	9.23
Housewife, retired, other	259	8.64	912	10.31	1171	9.94
Unemployed or student	64	10.98	127	11.64	191	11.42
Illness[a]						
No	307	6.61	382	8.35	689	7.58
Yes	705	8.52	1108	10.71	1813	9.86
Occupational Role[b]						
Worker	798	7.59	636	9.61	1434	8.49
Housewife	—	—	510	10.53	510	10.53
Retired	148	8.53	212	9.67	360	9.20
Umemployed	46	10.35	115	11.44	161	11.13
Student	20	12.00	17	12.41	37	12.19
Parental Status[a]						
Not living with children	288	6.81	477	9.15	765	8.27
Living with children	468	8.35	691	10.81	1159	9.82
No children	256	8.46	322	9.99	578	9.31

[a] One-way Analysis of variance overall $p < .02$ for both sexes.
[b] One-way analysis of variance, overall $p < .01$ for males; not significant for females.

both males and females, those who had had children but were not living with them ("empty nest" parents) were less depressed than others. Note that the average depression score for females was higher than that for males throughout Table 5.3, except among the high-level professionals. In some cases, however, the sex difference was quite small.

The same social factors were analyzed by sex separately for each marital status, to determine whether the sex-marital status interaction might be due to differences in these factors. In general, it can be seen that this is not the case. Adjusting for the social factors did not change the original findings of Table 5.2. Among the married (Table 5.4), the women were more depressed than the men except among the high-level and low-level professionals and the unemployed. Among the divorced-separated, Table 5.5 shows the women were more depressed than the men except in the sales and clerical occupations. Note however, that the few men in the survey living with children had average depression scores almost as high as the many women $N = (76)$ in that situation. Men and women who had exactly high school education also had very similar scores.

Among the never-married who were not heads of households, Table 5.6 shows the women were more depressed than men except among midlevel professionals, unskilled laborers, the "housewife, retired and other" occupational status category, the retired, and students. All of these groups contained very small numbers of people. However, the sex difference was not significant in any of these analyses, partly because of very unbalanced designs (small numbers in some cells). Table 5.7's data shows that among the never-married who were heads of household, it was usually the men who were more depressed, although not significantly so. The women were more depressed than the men only among those very small numbers of subjects with less than a high school education, or who were unemployed, students, or low-level professionals; and, reflecting very small differences, among the retired and those without illness. Again, none of the sex differences were significant.

Table 5.8 indicates that among the widowed, the men were also usually more depressed than the women. The women were more depressed than the men only among those with a high school or higher education (with small numbers of men and very small differences in mean scores) and among the small number of those working as laborers. The sex difference was significant ($p < .04$, with the men more depressed) only in the analysis by income, where numbers were reasonably balanced.

In summary, women were more depressed than men among the married and divorced-separated. Exceptions which seem interpretable were found in those married persons who were unemployed and divorced-separated people living with children. In the other groups, the sex dif-

TABLE 5.4
Average Depression Scores (CES-D) of Married Subjects by Sex and Other Social Factors

	MALE		FEMALE		TWO-WAY ANALYSIS OF VARIANCE	
	N	$\bar{X}$	*N*	$\bar{X}$		
Age					Sex × Age	$p = .510$
18–24	62	9.47	109	12.39	Sex	$p = .000$
25 & up	717	7.14	821	9.15	Age	$p = .000$
Education						
Less than high school	301	7.73	335	10.90	Sex × Education	$p = .095$
High school	254	7.78	360	9.61	Sex	$p = .000$
Beyond high school	224	6.25	235	7.46	Education	$p = .000$
Income					Sex × Income	$p = .728$
Less than $4000	68	9.32	84	11.01	Sex	$p = .004$
$4000 or more	669	7.20	775	9.35	Income	$p = .005$
Occupational Status						
High-level professional	38	5.58	4	3.25	Sex × Occupation	$p = .05$
Mid-level professional	88	5.86	41	7.66	Sex	$p = .09$
Low-level professional	92	7.37	23	7.35	Occupation	$p = .001$
Sales and Clerical	73	6.73	104	8.01		
Skilled manual	173	7.09	14	11.79		
Semi-skilled manual	82	9.01	56	9.91		
Unskilled manual	23	5.83	19	10.68		
Housewife, retired, other	179	7.46	586	9.95		
Unemployed or student	30	12.40	83	9.33		
Illness					Sex × Illness	$p = .72$
No	210	6.09	257	8.45	Sex	$p = .0001$
Yes	544	7.87	673	9.94	Illness	$p = .0003$
Occupational Role						
Worker	644	7.05	381	9.01	Sex × Occupation	$p = .01$
Retired	105	7.59	53	9.86	Sex	$p = .70$
Unemployed	24	12.79	77	9.40	Occupation	$p = .00$
Parental Status						
Not living with children	210	5.91	254	8.07	Sex × Parental status	$p = .51$
Living with children	458	8.21	571	10.14	Sex	$p = .0001$
No children	110	6.39	105	9.72	Parental status	$p = .0001$

ference was smaller and less consistent, with some tendency for men to be more depressed among the never-married heads of household and the widowed. The other social factors related to depression fairly consistently in all sex-marital status categories.

A variety of three-way analyses of variance were examined but they showed no dramatic departures from the patterns of Table 5.2. (The data are not shown on a table.) Analysis of covariance, using age, education, in-

TABLE 5.5
Average Depression Scores (CES-D) of Divorced-Separated Subjects, by Sex and Other Social Factors

	MALE		FEMALE		TWO-WAY ANALYSIS OF VARIANCE	
	N	x̄	*N*	x̄		
Age					Sex × Age	$p = .572$
18–24	4	12.25	17	20.82	Sex	$p = .019$
25 & up	62	7.61	128	12.80	Age	$p = .030$
Education						
Less than high school	25	7.28	74	14.86	Sex × Education	$p = .172$
High school	16	11.19	47	11.96	Sex	$p = .002$
Beyond high school	25	6.40	25	13.44	Education	$p = .721$
Income					Sex × Income	$p = .118$
Less than $4000	13	5.77	64	14.55	Sex	$p = .002$
$4000 or more	50	8.42	68	11.57	Income	$p = .926$
Occupational Status						
High-level professional	2	4.50	0	—	Omitting high level professionals	
Mid-level professional	6	7.33	11	11.45	Sex × Occupation	$p = .78$
Low-level professional	3	6.00	2	12.50	Sex	$p = .01$
Sales & clerical	5	12.40	29	11.93	Occupation	$p = .91$
Skilled manual	15	8.93	3	13.33		
Semi-skilled manual	5	9.60	24	11.33		
Unskilled manual	4	2.50	8	13.00		
Housewife, retired, other	19	6.74	55	15.47		
Unemployed or student	7	9.71	13	17.23		
Illness					Sex × Illness	$p = .23$
No	20	6.65	36	9.33	Sex	$p = .006$
Yes	46	8.43	109	15.16	Illness	$p = .02$
Occupational Role						
Worker	47	8.22	94	12.36	Sex × Occupation	$p = .42$
Retired	12	5.58	17	11.12	Sex	$p = .00$
Unemployed	5	6.20	11	17.53	Occupation	$p = .49$
Parental Status						
Not living with children	3	6.79	46	12.74	Sex × Parental status	$p = .53$
Living with children	6	14.17	76	14.70	Sex	$p = .08$
No children	17	8.47	23	12.39	Parental status	$p = .16$

come, occupational status, illness, and living with children as covariates, also did not change the pattern, although it reduced the sex difference in the divorced–separated and the never-married heads of household categories. For a description of regression analyses using a larger number of social factors, see Radloff and Rae (1979).

TABLE 5.6
Average Depression Scores (CES-D) of Never-Married (not Head of Household), Subjects by Sex and Other Social Factors

	MALE		FEMALE		TWO-WAY ANALYSIS OF VARIANCE	
	N	$\bar{x}$	*N*	$\bar{x}$		
Age					Sex × Age	$p = .564$
18–24	58	10.76	48	14.30	Sex	$p = .131$
25 & up	14	7.79	17	8.88	Age	$p = .007$
Education						
Less than high school	11	9.09	10	10.30	Sex × Education	$p = .597$
High school	37	9.57	27	13.59	Sex	$p = .143$
Beyond high school	24	11.63	24	12.92	Education	$p = .554$
Income					Sex × Income	$p = .793$
Less than $4000	5	11.20	5	12.40	Sex	$p = .526$
$4000 or more	55	9.98	41	12.49	Income	$p = .819$
Occupational Status						
High-level professional	0	–	0	–	Omitting high-level and low-level	
Mid-level professional	3	9.00	4	7.50	professionals	
Low-level professional	0	–	1	4.00	Sex × Occupation	$p = .33$
Sales & Clerical	4	10.50	9	12.11	Sex	$p = .58$
Skilled manual	9	6.44	1	10.00	Occupation	$p = .51$
Semi-skilled manual	11	8.82	7	14.43		
Unskilled manual	10	11.50	4	6.50		
Housewife, retired, other	19	12.63	19	12.58		
Unemployed or student	15	10.00	16	16.31		
Illness						
No	25	10.84	19	11.21	Sex × Illness	$p = .27$
Yes	46	9.96	42	13.50	Sex	$p = .17$
					Illness	$p = .63$
Occupational Role						
Worker	54	10.00	35	11.86		
Retired	2	17.00	4	12.00	Sex × Occupation	$p = .836$
Unemployed	10	8.00	8	18.75	Sex	$p = .600$
Student	5	14.00	8	13.88	Occupation	$p = .317$

A THEORETICAL MODEL OF DEPRESSION

The sex-marital status interaction and the relationship of social factors to depression suggest that the sex difference in depression is not due entirely to biological factors. Klerman and Weissman, in Chapter 4, have reviewed a variety of theories of depression and related them to possible explanations for the sex difference. The model presented here (see also

TABLE 5.7
Average Depression Scores (CES-D) of Never-Married (Head of Household) Subjects, by Sex and Other Social Factors

	MALE		FEMALE		TWO-WAY ANALYSIS OF VARIANCE	
	N	$\bar{x}$	*N*	$\bar{x}$		
Age					Sex × Age	$p = .976$
18–24	21	12.33	19	11.16	Sex	$p = .526$
25 & up	29	8.24	66	7.15	Age	$p = .010$
Education						
Less than high school	9	4.89	20	8.65	Sex × Education	$p = .017$
High school	13	16.38	25	7.12	Sex	$p = .185$
Beyond high school	28	8.61	42	8.07	Education	$p = .037$
Income					Sex × Income	$p = .501$
Less than $4000	14	10.36	25	9.88	Sex	$p = .666$
$4000 or more	32	10.31	53	7.51	Income	$p = .518$
Occupational Status						
High-level professional	5	7.60	1	1.00	Sex × Occupation	$p = .07$
Mid-level professional	3	8.00	11	6.00	Sex	$p = .65$
Low-level professional	2	4.50	4	12.00	Occupation	$p = .02$
Sales & Clerical	6	10.83	21	6.57		
Skilled manual	5	6.60	1	1.00		
Semi-skilled manual	8	9.38	4	5.75		
Unskilled manual	4	26.00	2	13.50		
Housewife, retired, other	7	10.86	40	8.10		
Unemployed or student	10	7.70	3	20.67		
Illness					Sex × Illness	$p = .12$
No	21	6.29	17	7.00	Sex	$p = .27$
Yes	30	12.33	70	8.16	Illness	$p = .02$
Occupational Role						
Worker	37	10.89	54	7.35	Sex × Occupation	$p = .028$
Retired	2	7.00	25	7.08	Sex	$p = .094$
Unemployed	4	6.00	2	22.50	Occupation	$p = .346$
Student	6	8.83	1	17.00		

Radloff & Rae, 1979) is closest to the "learned helplessness" explanation, but incorporates aspects of the behavioral and cognitive models, as well as a sequential "coping" model (McLean, 1976). It suggests that the sex difference in depression is related to the different learning histories of males and females, which result in different ways of coping with stress.

The epidemiologic or "disease" model assumes that the probability that an individual will develop a given disease depends on that individual's susceptibility to the disease and the exposure to the precipitating factors which initiate the disease. In the case of depression, both susceptibility and

TABLE 5.8
Average Depression Scores (CES-D) of Widowed Subjects, by Sex and Other Social Factors

	MALE		FEMALE		TWO-WAY ANALYSIS OF VARIANCE	
	N	$\bar{X}$	*N*	$\bar{X}$		
Age					Sex × Age	$p = .56$
18–64	13	15.38	108	11.22	Sex	$p = .14$
65 & up	32	11.76	161	9.65	Age	$p = .08$
Education						
Less than high school	29	15.38	171	10.56	Sex × Education	$p = .20$
High school	10	9.30	49	10.84	Sex	$p = .110$
Beyond high school	4	7.25	44	8.64	Education	$p = .774$
Income					Sex × Income	$p = .857$
Less than $4000	21	14.62	134	10.94	Sex	$p = .039$
$4000 or more	21	11.81	98	8.70	Income	$p = .126$
Occupational Status						
High-level professional	0	–	0	–	Omitting Occ. levels	
Mid-level professional	0	–	2	13.00	1,2,4	
Low-level professional	1	19.00	3	8.67	Sex × Occupation	$p = .63$
Sales and Clerical	0	–	18	8.56	Sex	$p = .81$
Skilled manual	4	11.50	3	14.33	Occupation	$p = .69$
Semi-skilled manual	2	6.00	9	15.56		
Unskilled manual	1	4.00	8	4.88		
Housewife, retired, other	35	13.09	212	10.16		
Unemployed or student	2	18.00	12	13.08		
Illness					Sex × Illness	$p = .57$
No	6	11.17	53	6.62	Sex	$p = .16$
Yes	39	13.03	214	11.16	Illness	$p = .17$
Occupational Role						
Worker	16	11.77	74	9.79	Sex × Occupation	$p = .89$
Retired	27	13.04	113	9.92	Sex	$p = .30$
Unemployed	1	21.00	13	14.31	Occupation	$p = .47$
Parental Status						
Not living with children	34	12.29	176	9.77	Sex × Parental status	$p = .68$
Living with children	3	20.00	41	12.22	Sex	$p = .10$
No children	8	12.13	50	10.38	Parental status	$p = .27$

precipitating factors may include both biological and social factors. It is here suggested that there is a component of susceptibility that is a learned habit, which could be called a "helpless style of coping," and that the precipitating factors which would activate this kind of susceptibility would be problems or stresses that need to be coped with.

General learning theory has shown that in the presence of a goal, such as obtaining a reward or avoiding a punishment, the response that succeeds in reaching the goal (i.e., is reinforced) will be "learned" (i.e., will be more likely to occur again in similar circumstances). In learning theory terms, this is known as learned instrumental behavior. The layman might call it "learning to cope." In humans, this learning may be accompanied by cognitions which could be verbalized: "In this situation, if I do this, that will happen."

Learning will not occur if any part of the sequence is absent, that is, if there is no goal, no response, no reinforcement, or no contingency between response and reinforcement. A person may not learn to cope if one or more of these factors is consistently missing. For example, extremely overprotected or "spoiled" children may learn as little as children in an extremely deprived environment. People cannot learn to obtain rewards by their own responses if rewards are either always or never available regardless of their actions, so that there is a lack of contingency. They may also fail to develop goals if they never want for anything or never have anything. If the person cannot or does not make the responses which would succeed in reaching a goal, lacking appropriate skills, there will be no learning. Or, if rewards or punishments are completely independent of a person's responses, what Seligman (1975) has called an "uncontrollable situation," the person may generalize this helplessness to new situations. This generalized "learned helplessness" is related to depression.

It is possible that a person can also learn to *not* cope, as well as fail to learn to cope. If successful responses which are rewarded are also consistently punished, the person will be in conflict and may try to solve it by avoiding the situation entirely—by, for example, giving up the goal. It is also possible that people can be directly taught not to cope by instruction or example, (e.g. discouragement or disparagement by significant others). Whatever its origin, failure to cope may lead to a generalized habit of not responding, even when there is a goal which could be reached by some possible response. Failure to cope may also be verbalized in helpless cognitions such as "nothing I do matters," "I can't cope," or "I can't do anything right." These expressions are characteristic of depression. Beck (1976) suggests that these cognitions are a basic cause of depression. McLean (1976) suggests that depression is the result of anticipation of chronic failure which is the result of feelings of lack of control resulting from repeated goal frustrations.

It is suggested here that the cognitive dimension of depression, the expectation that goals cannot be reached by any responses available to the person, is a basic factor in learned *susceptibility* to depression. Depression itself will not occur unless there is a goal actively present. In other words, the precipitating factors which activate the susceptibility are goals (rewards desired or punishments to be escaped or avoided). Given a goal situation and the expectation that nothing the person can do will influence the outcome, the person is unlikely to try to do anything. This lack of activity is like the motivational-behavioral dimension of depression. Depending on the environment and the generality of the helpless cognitions, such a person would be faced with more and more unescaped punishments and fewer and fewer rewards. This would result in pain, anxiety, sadness and lack of enjoyment—the affective dimension of depression. There is speculation and some evidence (Brenner, 1979) that the vegetative dimension of depression may follow from severe and prolonged affective disturbance.

Theoretically, then, depression develops sequentially, but in real life it is no doubt a vicious cycle. For example the inability to cope would strengthen the helpless cognitions and contribute to low self-esteem. The sleep and appetite disturbances would reduce energy level and aggravate the motivational-behavioral deficit. The sadness and apathy would interfere with social relationships, thereby reducing reinforcements still further. Depression would continue to deepen unless the cycle were interrupted. Intervention at any point in the cycle might be effective for treatment. But if this model has any validity, to prevent a relapse, the cognitive (susceptibility) dimension must be changed. Reduction in precipitating factors may also be necessary in cases where they are abnormally numerous or stressful.

APPLICATION OF THE MODEL TO THE SEX DIFFERENCE AND OTHER RISK FACTORS

The kinds of people who are most likely to be depressed include the young, the poor, and poorly educated (especially if female), those with low-status occupations, those with illness, the unemployed and students, women who are married or divorced–separated, the men who are never-married heads of households or widowed, and both sexes if they were never married but were not heads of households. Seligman (1975) has analyzed a variety of risk factors for depression, especially poverty and school failure, in terms of learned helplessness: "A child reared in . . . poverty will be exposed to a vast amount of uncontrollability [p. 159]." A background of poverty and poor education would reduce a person's chances of learning effective coping habits, and leave him or her more vulnerable to depression. Since past poverty and poor education are often correlated with current poverty and low-status occupations or unemployment, the high levels of depression in these groups is understandable. They would be more susceptible due to past experiences and also currently exposed to more precipitating factors (problems to be coped with).

Physical illness may be related to depression because it produces actual helplessness or at least feelings of loss of control. The high level of depression in the young, and especially among students, is more difficult to explain. It is supported by other recent surveys (Benfari, Beiser, Leighton, and Mertens, 1972; Berkman, 1971) and suicide rate data (Seiden, 1969). This age group may be faced with problems which are more difficult for them to solve than are the problems faced by older people. A recent survey (ISR, 1979) found a large increase from 1957 to 1976 in worry and anxiety in younger age groups. In discussions with the author, high school and college students expressed feelings of helplessness and lack of control. More work is needed to explore this issue.

The sex–marital-status patterns can be explained in several stages. First, as it will be shown, women are more likely to have more of the learned susceptibility to depression than men. Second, selectivity in marriage can be hypothesized, so that the less helpless women and the more helpless men would be most likely to stay unmarried long enough to become heads of their own households (see Bernard, 1973). Third, divorce and separation, especially if joined with poverty and responsibility for children, can be seen as stressful situations filled with precipitating factors for depression. Divorced–separated women would be both more susceptible (as are married women) and more likely to have children, low incomes and low-status jobs, or be unemployed. Finally, widowhood can be seen as a more stressful precipitant for men, because they have never been prepared to cope with it in either practical terms (by taking over domestic chores) or psychological terms. There are very few widowed males, and in this sense they are deviates from the norm.

Evidence that the learning history of women is more likely to lead to the component of susceptibility to depression, which is due to a lack of instrumental coping, has been reviewed elsewhere (Radloff & Monroe, 1978). Only a brief summary and a few examples will be given here.

The most plentiful evidence comes from studies of sex role stereotypes. Stereotypes reflect what we expect from people. Studies have consistently found that people expect females, even healthy, newborn babies, to be weaker, less able to get what they want by their own actions, and therefore more in need of help and protection than males. What people expect of a person is likely to influence the way they treat him or her and the way he or she behaves. There is evidence that girls are more likely to have things done *for* them, while boys are shown how to do things for themselves.

In the studies of childrearing practices reviewed by Maccoby and Jacklin (1974), only one consistent sex difference is found: The actions of boys more frequently *have consequences* than do the actions of girls. Granted, the boys are often punished especially for aggression, but both rewards and punishments depend on the boys' behavior. Boys can therefore learn to control rewards and punishments by their own actions. In contrast, an observational study of nursery schools (Serbin, O'Leary, Kent, & Tonick 1973) found that girls received fewer reactions from adults for all behaviors, including aggression. The authors describe, for example, a small girl who struck out aggressively in anger and was totally ignored. Even her worst temper tantrum had no effect on her environment. That is the ultimate in helplessness, and is reminiscent of clinical descriptions of the impotent rage of the angry depressive.

For males in our culture, achievement and competence are clearly rewarded. For females, they receive mixed results. Some studies found that females who displayed competence were simply ignored. For example, studies of small group problem-solving found that females were less listened to, were more often interrupted and had less influence on the group decisions. An extreme example is found in a study where females were given the right answer ahead of time, but still could not get the group to accept it (Altmeyer & Jones, 1974).

Other studies found that competent females sometimes got rewards, but were often also punished, especially by social rejection. The "fear of success" studies illustrate this. When a female was portrayed as successful, especially in achievement-oriented ways, people predicted many bad consequences of her success. In another study, male and female actors portrayed assertive and nonassertive roles. The assertive females were rated by observers as less likeable and more in need of psychotherapy than nonassertive females; the reverse was true for male actors (Costrich, Feinstein, Kidder, Marecek, and Pascale, 1975).

Other studies, (reviewed by Frieze, 1975) have found that females who succeeded in a task were more likely than males to attribute their success to luck or other factors which would not allow them to take credit for their achievement. This could produce a cognitive barrier to learning, by blocking the effectiveness of positive reinforcement. Females were less likely than males to expect to succeed in the future, and were less likely to *attempt* to succeed in the future. Recently, it has been found that depressed people are likely to have a similar "attribution style." When they do well at something, they attribute it to luck; when they fail, they take all the blame (Rizley, 1978). This attribution could be described as a generalized expectancy of failure to cope.

Many studies have found that work produced by females was rated as less significant, and was less rewarded by pay, promotions, and status than comparable work produced by men (e.g. see Huber, 1973; Safilios-Rothschild, 1972). "Women's work" is sometimes defined as "pleasing other people." Success in pleasing people is unpredictable, and the rewards are very intangible.

In summary, for "competent behavior" which, in our culture is highly praised, females, as compared to males, have been found to get fewer rewards, have less control over their rewards, and more often see their rewards accompanied by punishment, producing conflict, which interferes with learning. Women have also been instructed by the stereotypes that competent instrumental behavior is not expected of them. That this "training in helplessness" has been effective is shown by their attribution style–taking less personal credit for success—and their low expectations of success. The behavioral effect is seen in their reduced rates of attempting to solve problems.

It is suggested that depression is a special problem for women not because they are biologically female nor only because they are exposed to greater numbers of stress-inducing situations, but because they have learned to be more susceptible to depression. There are many sources of learned susceptibility which would affect both sexes equally, but stereotyped sex-role socialization is an added source of susceptibility to depression for women. The implications for treatment and prevention are obvious.

REFERENCES

Altemeyer, R., & Jones, K. Sexual identity, physical attractiveness and seating position as determinants of influence in discussion groups. *Canadian Journal of Behavior*, 1974, *6*, 357–375.

Beck, A. T. *Cognitive therapy and the emotional disorders.* New York: International Universities Press, 1976.

Benfari, R. C., Beiser, M., Leighton, A. & Mertens, C. Some dimensions of psychoneurotic behavior in an urban sample. *Journal of Nervous and Mental Diseases*, 1972, *155*(2), 77–90.

Berkman, P. L. Measurement of mental health in a general population survey. *American Journal of Epidemiology*, 1971, *94*, 105–111.

Bernard, J. *The future of marriage.* New York: Bantam Books, 1973.

Brenner, B. Depressed affect as a cause of associated somatic problems. *Psychological Medicine*, 1979, *9*, 737–746.

Comstock, G. W., & Helsing, K. J. Symptoms of depression in two communities. *Psychological Medicine*, 1976, *6*, 551–563.

Costrich, N., Feinstein, J., Kidder, L., Marecek, J., & Pascale, L. When stereotypes hurt: Three studies of penalties for sex-role reversals. *Journal of Experimental Social Psychology*, 1975, *11*, 520–530.

Frieze, I., Fisher, J. McHugh, M., & Valle, V. Attributing the causes of success and failure: Internal and external barriers to achievement in women. Paper presented at conference *New Directions for Research on Women*, Madison, Wisconsin, 1975.

Huber, J. (Ed), Changing women in a changing society. Chicago: University of Chicago Press, 1973.

Institute for Social Research Newsletter. Americans seek self-development, suffer anxiety from changing roles. *Institute for Social Research Newsletter.* The University of Michigan, 1979, *5*(winter), 4–5.

Maccoby, E. E., & Jacklin, C. N. *The Psychology of sex differences.* California: Stanford University press, 1974.

McLean, P. Therapeutic decision-making in behavioral treatment of depression. In Davidson, P. O. (Ed.), *The behavioral management of anxiety, depression and pain.* New York: Brunner/Mazel, 1976.

Radloff, L. S. Sex differences in depression: The effects of occupation and marital status. *Sex Roles,* 1975, *1*(3), 249–265.

Radloff, L. S. The CES-D scale: A self-report depression scale for research in the general population. *Journal of Applied Psychological Measurement,* 1977, *1,* 385–401.

Radloff, L. S. Depression and the empty nest. *Sex Roles,* in press.

Radloff, L. S., & Monroe, M. M. Sex differences in helplessness: With implications for depression. In Hansen, L. S., & Rapoza, R. S. (Eds.), *Career development and counselling of women.* Springfield, Ill.: Charles C Thomas, 1978.

Radloff, L. S., & Rae, D. S. Susceptibility and precipitating factors in depression: Sex differences and similarities. *Journal of Abnormal Psychology,* 1979, *88*(2), 174–181

Safilios-Rothschild (Ed) *Toward a sociology of women.* Lexington, Mass. Xerox Coll. 1972.

Rizley, R. Depression and distortion in the attribution of causality. *Journal of Abnormal Psychology,* 1978, *87,* 32–48.

Seiden, R. H. Suicide among youth: A review of the literature, 1900–1967. *The Bulletin of Suicidology,* National Institute of Mental Health, December 1969, 1–62.

Seligman, M. E. P. *Helplessness: On depression, development, and death.* San Francisco: W. H. Freeman, 1975.

Serbin, L. A., O'Leary, K. D., Kent, R. N., & Tonick, I. J. A comparison of teacher response to the preacademic and problem behavior of boys and girls. *Child Development,* 1973, *44,* 796–804.

Silverman, C. *The epidemiology of depression.* Baltimore: The Johns Hopkins Press, 1968.

Weissman, M. M., & Paykel, E. *The depressed woman: A study of social relationships.* Chicago: University of Chicago Press, 1974.

Weissman, M. M., Sholomskas, D., Pottenger, M., Prusoff, B. A., & Locke, B. Z. Assessing depressive symptoms in five psychiatric populations: A validation study. *American Journal of Epidemiology,* 1977, *106,* 203–214.

Chapter 6

STRESS AND THE MENTAL HEALTH OF WOMEN: A DISCUSSION OF RESEARCH AND ISSUES[1]

Vivian Parker Makosky

It almost goes without saying that women's mental health is related to the stress in their lives. We all "know" that. But when one attempts to document the relationship, or determine which stress-producing situations are really the critical ones for particular groups of women, or use the research literature as a basis for making policy recommendations relating to mental health services for women, it quickly becomes apparent that there are big gaps in the available information. In this chapter, I will outline some of the things we know, some of the things we do not know, and some of the things which need to be done in this area.

First, of course, it must be specified what is meant by the word "stress." The term has been used in a variety of ways (Dohrenwend & Dohrenwend 1974b), each with some justification. In this chapter, "stress" will be used broadly to mean a person's experience of upset, distress, discontent, discomfort, difficulty, adjustment, worry, concern, and so on. Thus, stress is being defined as an internal state of the person, which is in line with the early formulations of Selye and of Wolff (in Hinkle, 1974). At the same time, major emphasis is placed on the person's own appraisal of the situation relative to his or her well-being, rather than on the objective situation itself. This is a position on stress recently presented by Lazarus (1974), Hinkle (1974), and Thurlow (1971), among others. The event or condition which gives rise to stress is the "stressor." The "outcome" of being under stress—the response to stress, which is the focus of this chapter—is the increased likelihood of impaired functioning or illness. Although the

[1] The literature review was completed in January, 1977.

ISBN 0-12-310850-0

three entities stressors, stress, and outcomes, are conceptually distinct, they are often functionally circular. Stressors and outcomes of stress often overlap, as in the case of worry about a poor marital relationship, leading to impaired sexual functioning, which is, in turn, a source of increased stress. Although this circularity problem is a very important one to theorists, and to researchers who are trying to design "clean" studies, it is less important to policymakers and practitioners, because their primary focus is on the problem manifested, regardless of whether that problem is a stressor, an outcome of stress, or both.

SOME THINGS WE KNOW (Being Mostly Things We Knew We Know)

Practitioners have long noticed events or conditions in a person's life that are not directly harmful yet can contribute to the development of illness. Freud, for example, is famous (or infamous) for the emphasis he placed on the events of early childhood. As far back as the 1930s, at least, Adolph Meyer advocated the use of a life chart in medical diagnosis, and suggested that it should include not only the medical history of the patient, but also such events as births, deaths, moves, job changes, graduations, and so forth. (Winters [1951]). Others emphasize different events, conditions, or periods in the life cycle as important (Klerman & Izen, 1974; Money & Ehrhardt, 1974; Seidenberg, 1975). In some cases, the assertions have been speculative, based on years of personal clinical experience rather than upon experimentation or other formal research procedures. Nevertheless, subsequent research has supported a number of early assertions and has further refined our understanding of these relationships.

Meyer's teachings about the use of a life chart in medical diagnosis rested on the assumption that life changes—even "good" ones—may be hazardous to one's health. This assumption also underlies the research tools developed by Holmes and Rahe (1967) and their colleagues. Three of their tools use the same list of 43 life events, some positive and some negative. The Social Readjustment Rating Questionnaire gives instructions for scaling each item in terms of the average amount of adjustment that that event would require of the subject. The Social Readjustment Rating Scale assigns adjustment scores to each life event, resulting in a summary of the *life-change units* a subject reports. The Schedule of Recent Experiences, a self-administered questionnaire, has the respondent record those life events for the preceding 10 years, and allows the researcher to assign total life-change units for various periods of time within that 10-year span. The steps in the development of these instruments and a summary of some of the relevant research findings are presented in Holmes and Masuda (1974). These tools, which allow systematic measurement and quantification of life changes, have been a major force in determining the direction of life stress research, both within medicine and in other disciplines. The magnitude of the influence exerted is plain from the work presented in two recent books, *Stressful life events: Their nature and effects* (Dohrenwend & Dohrenwend, 1974a) and *Life stress and illness* (Gunderson & Rahe, 1974).

An inspection of these two volumes gives a broad overview of relevant research findings. In terms of *physical* illness, they summarize a number of studies which point to the relationship between a clustering of life events and subsequent general illness behavior (days of work missed, seeking of medical aid, etc.), as well as between event clusters and the onset of such specific syndromes as tuberculosis, heart disease, skin disease, hernia, bone fractures, transient diabetes, and leukemia in children. Outside the realm of physical illness, clustering of life events has been found to precede incarceration in a federal prison, pregnancy, decline in academic performance, and the decline in work performance of high school teachers. The situation with regard to *mental health* is ably summarized by Hudgens (1974):

> As I interpret the results of recent studies, . . . investigators have demonstrated a causal connection between stressful life events and subsequent worsening of conditions already under way, between life events and subsequent admission to psychiatric hospitals or clinics, and in a substantial minority of bereaved persons, between bereavement and depression of moderate degree for which psychiatric care was rarely sought. It does not seem to me that investigators have yet convincingly demonstrated that life stress can cause madness in a person previously of sound mind, nor can it cause severe depression sustained for many months and attended by multiple disturbance [sic] of physical and mental function [p. 120].

In particular, a clustering of life events, or of particular types of life events, are reported as preceding suicide, depression, and schizophrenia (e.g., Brown, 1974; Coleman, 1973; Paykel, 1974a,b); and a high life change unit score and/or clustering of events are related to depressed mood and to psychophysiologic symptoms in the general population (Markush & Favero, 1974; Myers, Lindenthal, & Pepper, 1974; Dohrenwend, 1973b).

A great deal of time and effort has been devoted to delineating what events are stressful, how stressful they are, and what the outcomes of this stress are. Some of the conclusions are that, by and large, negative events are more stressful than positive events (Paykel, 1974b); the same events are more stressful when they are recent than when they have receded into the past (Horowitz, Schaefer & Cooney, 1974); events in general tend to cluster in the 3 weeks just prior to the onset of schizophrenia or depression, but the clustering of moderately or markedly threatening events before the onset of depression extends over a period of at least 38 weeks (Brown, 1974); and events with long-term implications of threat are more stressful than those without such implications (Brown, 1974). Currently, work is being done (Dohrenwend, 1976) to relate the desirability of events to the person's ability to anticipate and/or control the event.

And so the work goes on. Unfortunately, it seems to be going on in the same vein, and not really addressing the problems that plague life-events research. For a good general critique of the work to date, see Rabkin and Struening (1976). For somewhat more limited critiques, see Mechanic (1974) or Dohrenwend (1974).

SOME THINGS WE DO NOT KNOW (Being Practically Everything That Is Relevant)

As in so many other areas of research, the study of sex differences in responses to life stress has been underemphasized. The two volumes *Stressful life events: Their nature and effects* and *Life stress and illness* have been warmly received within the sciences. For example, Horowitz (1975) said: "These volumes together are the vital texts on the currently powerful issue of the correlation between stressful life events and the onset of physical or psychological illness [p. 851]." Yet each volume had only one listing under "sex differences" or "effects of sex" in the topical index; and there were no listings for "women," "sex comparisons," or related headings. The research populations included in the studies were frequently exclusively or predominantly male: Prisoners of war, football players, industrial employees, medical interns, physicians, and Navy personnel at sea, for example. The sex of some populations was unspecified or mixed without a breakdown of analyses by sex. A few studies reported used female subjects only, but these were relatively scarce. Sex *comparisons* are largely unreported, so that we do not know whether the findings apply to men, to women, or to both. For example, Brown (1974) draws conclusions about differences in the clustering of life events preceding schizophrenia and depression, but those conclusions may be invalid because of the confounding of diagnosis and sex of subjects: the schizophrenic group included both females and males (no sex comparisons reported), whereas the depressed group was exclusively female.

Of course, it is always legitimate to ask whether there is any point to making sex comparisons—any reason to expect sex differences—and the answer in this instance is a resounding "yes." There is good evidence that the sexes differ in their patterns of mental health and/or illness (e.g., Bernard, 1973; Gurin, Veroff, & Feld, 1960; Guttentag & Salasin, 1976; Guttentag *et al.*, 1976; Uhlenhuth, Lipman, Balter, and Stern, 1974). Although much of the life stress research has used physical illness as the measured outcome, many times the illnesses were chronic syndromes, such as ulcers or heart disease, syndromes most frequently thought to be associated with life stress, and in which there are well-known sex differences in incidence (cf. Coleman, 1973). There is at least some evidence that women and men respond differently to the same psychosocial stressors. Langner and Michael (1963) report that in a normal population, although there was no sex difference in functional impairment, women reported a *greater* number of psychoneurotic and psychophysiological symptoms than did men; and when faced with money, work, or marital worries, women had a *greater* increment in risk for mental illness than did men. But more recently, Pearlin (1975a) reported that women are *less* depressed than men are by the same job strains. Of course, this contradiction in findings may be more apparent than real, because each study used a different measure of stress and a different measure of outcome. Although neither study was concerned with life-events lists, each purported to be dealing with stress, and each found differing responses among men and women. Obviously, additional information is needed to reach a conclusion.

As mentioned, sex comparisons in the study of life-events stressors and mental health are few. And those which exist indicate that here, too, more research is needed. One of the earliest references to relevant sex comparison in life events research is in Dohrenwend (1973b), a study using a checklist of life events for the preceding 12 months and ratings of life change based on the Social Readjustment Rating Scale of Holmes and Rahe (1967). Dohrenwend found that women had significantly higher life-change scores and significantly higher scores on Langner's 22-Item Scale of psychiatric symptoms than did men. When the effect of sex was controlled, there was still a significant correlation between life-change scores and psychological symptom scores. Women's symptom levels were more affected by events they did not control (such as illness of a loved one) than by the total of all events, whereas men's symptom scores were more closely related to their total life-change scores. Unfortunately, what seem to be nice, clearcut results have not been completely supported by the findings of others. Markush and Favero (1974) also use a general population sample, and they report that less educated, younger, and female subjects tended to have higher proportions of high depressed mood scores on the Center for Epidemiologic Studies Depression Scale (the CES-D Scale); women generally had a greater proportion of high scores on Langner's 22-Item Scale of symptoms; high depressed mood scores and high symptom scores were both related to high life-change unit scores. However, men and women did *not* have significantly different life-change unit scores. These findings are supported by those of Uhlenhuth *et al.* (1974), who also find that women and those with high life-stress scores, as assessed by total standard values assigned to 41 life events, had higher symptom intensities. But once again, there was no significant sex difference in life-stress scores.

Finally, in a study with a slightly different approach, Radloff (1974) compared the depression scores (on the CES-D Scale) for married working men, married working women, married housewives, never-married working men and never-married working women who had 0, 1 or 2+ life-event losses. She found that married working men were significantly less depressed than *any* of the other groups, at all levels of life event losses. In addition, the married working women were less depressed than the married housewives. Otherwise, the only significant differences were that as life events losses went up, so did depression scores.

To summarize, then, we know that life events, or particular life events, are related to high depression scores and to high levels of psychophysiological symptoms. We know that as a group, women have higher depression scores and higher levels of psychophysiological symptoms than do men. What we do *not* know is whether there is a consistent relationship between sex and life events stress.

What might account for these findings? There are three possible explanations. First, it may be that there are more stressors in the lives of women than in the lives of men, but the contents of the life-events lists do not reflect this. Second, the stressors may be the same, but women may experience greater stress than do men, which is not reflected in the scaling of the life events. And, third, the stressors and stress both may be comparable, but the sexes may *respond* differently, although this is not reflected in the life events studies to date. Radloff (1975) has generated a similar list of alternative explanations, based upon her own work and a review of a somewhat different body of research. Let us turn now to the evidence supporting each of these possible explanations.

The first explanation relates to a general issue raised by others (e.g., Dohrenwend, 1974; Rabkin & Struening, 1976), and that should be considered in conjunction with the discussion of stress and women's mental health: What life events are to be included within a study? Although there are certain similarities between the lists of 43 life events generated by Holmes and his colleagues and the lists used by other researchers, the overlap is general; the lists actually differ in length, wording, content, and emphasis. One cannot hope to either compile or use an exhaustive list of possible life events, and so the sampling of the universe of items is of primary importance. The selection of items for inclusion in most of the life-event lists to date may have served to underestimate the stressors in women's lives. For example, life-event lists typically ask a number of questions about work (whether one has been promoted, demoted, fired, changed work conditions or hours, had trouble with supervisor or coworkers, etc.) All of the events of this type would apply to a larger proportion of men than women. At the same time, the instructions typically ask about these work events in one's *own* life, and do not allow for the stresses in one's life caused by work events in the *spouse's* life—which would probably be greater for women. The only author found who mentioned this issue at all was Wilkins (1974), who said, "This *contagion of stress,* from husband to wife, is widely appreciated, but hardly tested in a scientific sense [p. 250]." He was referring specifically to work or economic stressors. Although neither he nor anyone else mentioned "contagion of stress" from wife to husband, the only item which might tap such a stressor on the Holmes and Rahe (1967) Schedule of Recent Events is "*Wife* starting or ending work"!

The concept of a contagion of stress is an important but thorny one. The authors of the various life-events lists have recognized it implicitly if not explicitly by including items related to the illness, injury, engagement, or marriage of family members and/or friends, and one sometimes finds "pregnancy of wife" or "birth of child (for father)" listed separately. However, the stress effects of events in the lives of significant others have not been studied systematically, and the absence of such contagion of stress items (particularly in the areas of work and money) have resulted in lists which systematically underestimate the stress in women's lives. The only bit of evidence related to this assertion is indirect, but telling. Dohrenwend (1976), in research which has a very different focus, asks subjects whether the events listed had happened, during the past 12 months, to them, to members of their families, or to other people who were important to them. She reports that there was a large sex difference in the proportion of reported events in which the interviewee was not the central figure. Many more of the events reported by women were things which had happened to family or friends. This finding takes on additional importance when considered in conjunction with an earlier finding (Dohrenwend, 1973b) that women's psychological symptom scores were determined more by events they did *not* control (i.e., things which happened to others) than by the total of all events; this was not true for men. Thus, it would seem that the majority of life-events studies to date have excluded a larger proportion of the events relevant to women than to men.

Besides not including items and instructions to accurately assess the contagion of stress in women's lives, life-events studies exclude a number of areas of direct stress as well. Some events which come immediately to mind include abortion, rape, physical assault, changes in childcare arrangements, and incidents of sex discrimination. Although some of these events would be less likely to be relevant to men than to women, the reverse has long been true of the items already in use, such as the items dealing with work and the draft. At the same time, as Dohrenwend (1974) points out, what constitutes a "common" life event varies tremendously depending on whether the population is one of old people, felons, psychiatric patients, or community leaders, and so on. I would simply add "women or men" to the list. It may be that there is no one list of common life events with comparable impacts on different people.

Another "content" issue which has been mentioned by others (e.g., Kellman, 1974; Rabkin & Struening, 1976; Wilkins, 1974), and is particularly relevant to the present discussion, is that the event lists generated to date all deal with "personal" events even though it is recognized that "[c]hanges caused by widespread social processes also heighten the individual's vulnerability to stress and stress-related diseases . . . (Rabkin & Struening, 1976, p. 1014)." The women's movement and changing sex roles within our society are cases in point. For at least some women, these concepts are the source of a significant amount of stress (McBride, 1976), but have not been systematically investigated in that context.

All in all, there is adequate cause to suspect that the item content of the events lists used in life-stress research is constructed in such a way as to produce misleading and inaccurately low life-change and/or stress scores for women. However, that is not the only source of possible bias. There is also a question as to whether the same stressors result in the same amount of stress for women and men.

Much of the research uses one of the instruments for assessing life change discussed by Holmes and Masuda (1974). Therefore, the scaling procedures used in deriving their standard life-change units for the various events should be examined. Although Holmes and Masuda (1974) report that the relative order and magnitude of the life events scaled were highly correlated for males and females in the sample (Pearson's $r = .965$), a sex biasing of weights is still a possibility. Subjects were asked to scale the events in terms of the *average* degree of readjustment necessary for each event (Holmes & Rahe, 1967); similarly, Paykel, Prusoff, and Uhlenhuth (1971), in deriving the scores which were used for the Uhlenhuth *et al.* (1974) study, asked subjects to try to think how upsetting the event would be to the *average person.* When Broverman, Broverman, Clarkson, Rosenkrantz, and Vogel (1970) asked raters about a man, a woman, or a person whose sex was unspecified, they found that the characteristics of a mentally healthy man and a person were the same, but that a mentally healthy woman was rated significantly differently from either of the others. Thus, there is some reason to suspect that ratings about average people might be biased in the direction of male values, possibly leading to artificially low change–stress scores for women. In addition, Holmes and Rahe (1967) subjects were told that marriage had been given an arbitrary value of 500 (the middle score), and they were asked to rate all other events in terms of whether they required more or less readjustment than marriage. It is quite possible that marriage, on the average, causes more change in the lives of women than of men, and that the rates therefore had a discrepant constant which skewed the final values. Although groups of different ages, classes or subcultures have done event scaling, the studies have nearly all included instructions concerning the average person and/or have used potentially biased anchor events. A study by Rosenberg and Dohrenwend (1975) finds significant differences in the ratings of the readjustment necessitated by marriage depending on the ethnic background and experience of the raters, but *no* sex differences. However, the authors do not describe their instructions to subjects in the published report.

The one published report that neither used an anchor nor asked about an average person was by Horowitz *et al.* (1974), in which subjects were asked to imagine how much "stress" they would be under at the present time if the specified event had occurred one week ago, one month ago, six months ago, one year ago, or three years ago. These authors divided their 34 items into seven logical sets: major deaths, important separations, arguments with important persons, major threats to self or self-image, moderate to minor threats to self or self-image, threats to material well-being, and general change without negative connotations. In this study, women rated all logical sets as significantly more stressful than did men at the one-week time interval; at the three-year time interval, the only other interval for which results were given, women still rated major threats to self as significantly more stressful than did men. There were no comparisons reported on which *men* rated the stress to be greater than did the women. Seidenberg (1975) maintains that changing residence, especially moving to another city or state, is more traumatic for women. And if we extend the position of Brown (1974), that events with a longer-term threat are more stressful, then we can readily build the case that separation, divorce, widowhood, and childbearing (among others) are more stressful events for women than for men, because women are likely to suffer greater financial loss, are less likely to remarry, and are more likely to have the care of the children, regardless of marital status.

So although there is little direct evidence of greater stress of particular life events for women, it certainly seems possible that that is the case, and that assigning the same readjustment or stress values to events for both men and women distorts the relationships. This suggestion certainly bears further investigation. Comparison of results of tests using different instructions would be one good way of approaching the problem.

The point of this discussion is that the content and scaling of life-events lists may have systematically underestimated the amount of stress in women's lives related to life changes. But even if the content and scaling problems were corrected, the resulting standard score would still be only a reflection of the average, or group norm for each event. Although a valid average rating would suffice for large-scale, group comparisons, it would still mask the wide range of individual differences in responses to particular life events. Some researchers have also recognized this problem and have attempted to deal with it in a number of ways. Brown (1974) describes a system wherein four investigators met to discuss the meaning of given events in the context of a particular person's life, and assigned a consensus rating of the severity of threatening implications. In making these ratings, the investigators went to some lengths to discount the subject's *own* assessment of the impact of the event. Pearlin (1975a, 1975b) uses a self-report measure of stress, and Bronfenbrenner (1976) is in the initial stages of a study which will use a self-report measure of stress, but neither of these investigators is working in the context of life-events research. Rahe (1974) reports that his research unit is experimenting with a method for obtaining a subjective life-change unit scaling system which asks subjects the amount of readjustment, based on both the intensity and the duration of the readjustment, required by each of the scale's life events that they have experienced. However, at the time of this writing, reports of research using those instructions were not available. Such a system would have disadvantages, of course, particularly with regard to report bias, distortion of recall, and so forth. Only empirical work, however, can determine whether the "objective" or "subjective" estimate of stress is the better predictor of subsequent illness.

If all of the suggestions for additional research were acted upon, we would still not have eliminated the third possible source of sex differences thus far reported in the literature: The possibility that even when men and women experience the same *amount* of stress, they respond differently.

The data relating to sex differences in outcomes of stressful life events are few. Radloff (1974, 1975) reports that working married men, the group least likely to respond to life events losses with depression, also had no apparent alternate response or compensation for depression. They were not consistently higher than the other groups in physical illness, psychophysiological symptoms, aggression, poor social functioning, or alcoholism. She concludes, on the basis of her data and a review of work by others, that what is needed is additional investigation of such resources as self-esteem, social supports, education, and income (Radloff, 1974).

There seems to have been little life-events research dealing with sex differences in coping and/or support systems. No studies were found that use life-events checklists and also report on coping and/or support systems.

However, there are studies relating life crises or a particular life event to coping. The typical approach has been to operationally define the high-stress group as one which has had a particular, unquestionably stressful experience, often what one would term a crisis. Such operational definitions have included, for example, having survived an earthquake, incarceration in a concentration camp, combat, or a prisoner-of-war experience. When those who have experienced these crises are compared with those who have not, it is found that the former show a much higher proportion of physical and psychological problems, lasting anywhere from a few days to years after the experience (e.g., Arthur, 1974; Coleman, 1973). In these studies there is usually no attempt to quantify the amount of stress experienced; a dichotomous state of high stress versus low stress (rather than a continuum) is assumed. Then, too, these experiences are far from the "normal" events that people experience. For these reasons, this research has only a small degree of relevance to the present discussion. One of the most impressive things about the life crisis research is the near universality of observable negative outcomes, regardless of prior adjustment of the individual, or other factors (Arthur, 1974; Dohrenwend, 1975). However, although it seems that no one is immune to negative outcomes, there are people who show fewer and/or less severe outcomes. These people differ from the rest of the group by showing a certain emotional insensitivity, which at least some researchers have classified as a coping mechanism (Hinkle, 1974).

About half of the articles on life stress reviewed have made some mention of coping and/or support systems, often with some suggestion for what they might be or how they might work (e.g., Antonovsky, 1974; Coleman, 1973; Kagan & Levi, 1974; Lazarus, 1974; Nelson, 1974; Rabkin & Struening, 1976). But, once again, little of this directly relates to the topic here discussed. Lazarus (1974) mentions denial and detachment as effective coping strategies for the parents of a child dying of leukemia, combat air crews, patients with severe burns, paralytic polio victims, surgical patients, and terminally ill cancer patients, among others. Hinkle (1974) cites emotional insulation as a factor in minimizing the effects of "objectively" stressful events. Pearlin (1975b), on the other hand, emphasizes active coping as the best strategy for dealing with stress of marital or parental origin, and considers intrapsychic coping (psychological defenses) to be, in general, the least effective way of dealing with stress of economic or occupational origin. He reports that for each of the four areas of stress mentioned, selective ignoring was the least effective technique. At the same time, an optimistic outlook—expecting things to get better in the next year or two, and considering oneself to be as well or better off than one's peers—did a lot to minimize what might otherwise have been the depressive consequences of an objectively bad situation for women (Pearlin, 1975a). These coping strategies were studied in very limited contexts; none were in the context of quantified life-events stressors, and most were intrapsychic defense mechanisms, rather than coping strategies of a more direct-action type, such as discussing one's marital problems with one's spouse (a distinction made by Lazarus, 1974). No study reported sex differences. At the very least, however, the data tend to support the assertion that different sources of stress may call for different methods of coping. For example, if there is a serious problem that cannot be overcome, it may be best to try to ignore it. If the dilemma is amenable to change, however, active steps might prove more effective. Obviously, this issue also needs more work, especially in the areas of quantifiable life stress of identifiable origin and the utility of a variety of coping mechanisms.

In terms of the usefulness of social supports, there are some data relevant to women's mental health. A study of pregnant women by Nuckolls, Cassell, and Kaplan (1972) demonstrates that the higher risk of complications of later pregnancy and delivery associated with high life change was mitigated by social supports. Ninety percent of the women with high life-change scores and low social-support scores had pregnancy complications, while only 33% of those with high life-change scores and high social-support scores had complications. Similarly, Brown, Bhrolchain, and Harris (1975) conclude that intimacy acts as a powerful mediator between stressors and psychiatric disturbance. Although Pearlin (1975b) does not find that seeking help or advice from others was effective in dealing with marital, parental, economic, or occupational stress, he also reports (1975a) that when women are separated from a network of social relationships, they are more likely to be disenchanted with the homemaker role. Rabkin and Struening (1976) conclude that although social support systems are irrelevant when a person is not under stress, the lack of such systems may exacerbate the outcomes of stress when stressful situations exist.

In a discussion of life stress and mental health, coping mechanisms and support systems are extremely important because they mitigate negative outcomes of stress, presumably by ameliorating the person's feeling of stress. The failure to take into account the coping and support resources of the people confronted by life-event stressors may be one of the primary reasons for the low correlations reported to date between lists of stressful life events and illness outcomes. As Rabkin and Struening (1976) point out, there are many weaknesses in the statistical treatment of life-events research. Most of the correlations reported range between .12 and .30. When this is the case, the relationships established may be statistically significant but practically useless. Indeed, when low correlations are obtained with group data, the data are not very useful in making predictions in individual cases. What these low correlations signify is that there are wide individual differences in responses to life stressors, and that more emphasis needs to be placed on the exploration of relevant mediating variables, such as coping mechanisms and social support systems. However, other factors might also affect one's feeling of stress, and thus, presumably, the outcomes of being exposed to stressors.

One more area in which more information is needed is the area of stressful life *conditions.* The primary emphasis in this chapter, and in much of the research, has been on stressful life *events.* As already mentioned, the general relationships reported tend to be reliable but weak. Part of the reason for this may be that events are only one general type of stressor in a person's life, and that much of the meaning of an event depends on the conditions which form the context of that event. Support for this position is apparent, not only intuitively, but also from research. There is a large body of literature indicating that the following life conditions, at least, are related to one's mental health and/or illness: age, sex, marital status, race, work status, social class, parental status, residential location, minority status, and social isolation (Bernard, 1973; Dohrenwend & Dohrenwend, 1972; Dohrenwend, 1975; Garai, 1970a & b; Gurin *et al.*, 1960; Guttentag & Salasin, 1975; Langner & Michael, 1963; Myers *et al.*, 1974; Pearlin & Johnson, 1975; Rabkin & Struening, 1976; Radloff, 1975). As some of the work cited earlier shows, these conditions not only have an effect on mental health, but they interact with each other as well. And that is the difficulty when it comes to relating stressful life events to stressful life conditions. Although each of these conditions has been related in one way or another to life-events research, they are typically considered one at a time. The study by Radloff (1974, 1975) in which she relates life-event losses to sex, work status, *and* marital status, is an outstanding exception. But even in that study, these life conditions were used as classification variables, and it is apparent that there is a limit—a low limit—on the number of sorting variables which can be applied simultaneously. Stressful life conditions should be *quantified,* so that an additive score could be obtained reflecting the additional magnitude of the stressor. For example, one could have a financial stressor score based not only on income level (a typical classification variable), but also on predictability, variability, fixed expenses, etc.

Brown *et al.* (1975) relates life events and long-term difficulties in housing, money, children, health, and marriage to psychiatric disturbance in women. They find that events and major difficulties both play a causal role in depression. In addition, they use a crude four-point scale of vulnerability based on intimacy, age and number of children at home, employment status, and whether the respondent had lost her mother in childhood. They find that "The proportion with an onset (of psychiatric disturbance) among those with an event or difficulty ranges from 6 percent for those with a score of 0 or 1, 45 percent for 2, and 100 percent for 3 or more [p. 239]." The basis for distinguishing between difficulties and vulnerability factors was not clear from the published report, and both could be classified as stressful life conditions. However, the study does give support to the position that events *and* conditions are relevant, and that conditions can be quantified. In short, some of the stress in one's life is not related to how much things are changing, but to how persistent an oppressive condition is. The whole area of quantifying stressful life conditions, considering both their severity and duration, is in need of development.

Another area which should be investigated is the breadth of outcomes resulting from exposure to stressors, particularly in the general population. The measures used to date (e.g., the CES-D Scale, the Gurin *et al.* (1960) items,; and the Langner 22-Item Scale) are closely related to measures of anxiety (Gersten, Langner, Eisenberg, & Orzek, 1974). Although anxiety measures are perfectly legitimate measures, more variety is needed—specifically, more work using measures of role functioning (work, marital, parental, social), aggression, antisocial behavior, and drug dependency.

SOME THINGS THAT NEED TO BE DONE

There is ample evidence that life stress and physical and mental health are related, but not enough information about how they are related for women. Thus, we need to try alternative lists of life-events items, and alternative scaling procedures, to assess their applicability for women. We need to isolate more clearly the source of stress, rather than lumping all life events together, and include not only events but also conditions. Greater specificity would yield a much more useful diagnostic tool. In addition, if data were gathered concerning the social supports and coping mechanisms available and useful to individual women or groups of women, we would be in a better position to help them deal with the outcomes of stress. Finally, we need reliable measurement tools for quantifying *both* the objective stressors (events or conditions in the woman's life) and also the subjective stress (the feelings of upset reported by the woman herself). Were all of this done, we would be able to make a much stronger case for the ways in which events and conditions in the lives of individual women and groups of women are related to their mental health. On that basis we could make informed recommendations concerning public policy and social intervention programs, as well as help individual women in the most effective way possible.

REFERENCES

Antonovsky, A. Conceptual and methodological problems in the study of resistance resources and stressful life events. In Dohrenwend, B. S., & Dohrenwend, B. P. (Eds.), *Stressful life events: Their nature and effects.* New York: Wiley, 1974.

Arthur, R. J. Extreme stress in adult life and its psychic and psychophysiological consequences. In Gunderson, E. K. E., & Rahe, R. H., *Life stress and illness.* Springfield, Ill.: Charles C Thomas, 1974.

Bernard, J. *The future of marriage.* New York: Bantam Books, 1973.

Bronfenbrenner, U. Conceptual framework, section F categories for assessing parental stresses and supports. Personal communication, September 22, 1976.

Broverman, I. K., Broverman, D. M., Clarkson, F. E., Rosenkrantz, P. S., & Vogel, S. Sex-role stereotypes and clinical judgments of mental health. *Journal of Consulting and Clinical Psychology,* 1970, *34*(1), 1–7.

Brown, G. W. Life-events and the onset of depressive and schizophrenic conditions. In Gunderson, E. K. E., & Rahe, R. H., *Life stress and illness.* Springfield, Ill.: Charles C Thomas, 1974.

Brown, G. W., Bhrolchain, M. N., & Harris, T. Social class and psychiatric disturbance among women in an urban population. *Sociology,* 1975, *9,* 225–254.

Coleman, J. C. Life stress and maladaptive behavior. *The American Journal of Occupational Therapy,* 1973, *27*(4), 169–180.

Dohrenwend, B. P. Problems in defining and sampling the relevant population of stressful life events. In Dohrenwend, B. S., & Dohrenwend, B. P. (Eds.), *Stressful life events: Their nature and effects.* New York: Wiley, 1974.

Dohrenwend, B. P. Sociocultural and social-psychological factors in the genesis of mental disorders. *Journal of Health and Social Behavior,* 1975, *16*(4), 365–392.

Dohrenwend, B. S. Anticipation and control of stressful life events: An exploratory analysis. Paper presented at the Eastern Psychological Association Convention, New York, 1976.

Dohrenwend, B. S. Life events as stressors: A methodological inquiry. *Journal of Health and Social Behavior,* 1973, *14,* 167–175. (a)

Dohrenwend, B. S. Social status and stressful life events. *Journal of Personality and Social Psychology,* 1973, *28*(2), 225–235. (b)

Dohrenwend, B. S., & Dohrenwend, B. P. A brief historical introduction to research on stressful life events. In Dohrenwend, B. S., & Dohrenwend, B. P. (Eds.), *Stressful life events: Their nature and effects.* New York: Wiley, 1974. (b)

Dohrenwend, B. S., & Dohrenwend, B. P. Social class and the relation of remote to recent stressors. In Roff, M., Robins, L. N., & Pollack, M. (Eds.), *Life history research in psychopathology* (Vol. 2). Minneapolis: University of Minnesota Press, 1972.

Dohrenwend, B. S., & Dohrenwend, B. P. (Eds.) *Stressful life events: Their nature and effects.* New York: Wiley, 1974. (a)

Garai, J. E. Sex differences in identity and intimacy. *Genetic Psychology Monographs,* 1970, *81*(2), 133–134. (a)

Garai, J. E. Sex differences in the breakdown of mental health. *Genetic Psychology Monographs,* 1970, *81*(2), 131–132. (b)

Gersten, J. C., Langner, T. S., Eisenberg, J. G., & Orzek, L. Child behavior and life events: Undesirable change or change *per se*? In Dohrenwend, B. S., & Dohrenwend, B. P. (Eds.), *Stressful life events: Their nature and effects.* New York: Wiley, 1974.

Gunderson, E. K. E., & Rahe, R. H. *Life stress and illness.* Springfield, Ill.: Charles C Thomas, 1974.

Gurin, G., Veroff, J., & Feld, S. *Americans view their mental health.* New York: Basic Books, 1960.

Guttentag, M., & Salasin, S. Women, men and mental health. In Carter, L., Scott, A., & Martyna, W. *Women and men: Changing roles and perceptions.* New York: Aspen Institute for Humanistic Studies, 1976.

Guttentag, M., Salasin, S., Legge, W., Bray, H., Dewhirst, J., Goldman, N., Phegley, T., & Weiss, S. Sex differences in the utilization of publicly supported mental health facilities: The puzzle of depression. Unpublished manuscript, 1976.

Hinkle, L. E., Jr. The concept of "stress" in the biological and social sciences. *International Journal of Psychiatry in Medicine,* 1974, *5*(4), 335–357.

Holmes, T. H., & Masuda, M. Life change and illness susceptibility. In Dohrenwend, B. S., & Dohrenwend, B. P. (Eds.), *Stressful life events: Their nature and effects.* New York: Wiley, 1974.

Holmes, T. H., & Rahe, R. H. The social readjustment rating scale. *Journal of Psychosomatic Research,* 1967, *11,* 213–218.

Horowitz, M. J., Schaefer, C., & Cooney, P. Life event scaling for recency of experience. In Gunderson, E. K. E., & Rahe, R. H., *Life stress and illness.* Springfield, Ill.: Charles C Thomas, 1974.

Horowitz, M. J. New directions in epidemiology. *Science,* 1975, *188,* 850–851.

Hudgens, R. W. Personal catastrophe and depression: A consideration of the subject with respect to medically ill adolescents, and a requiem for retrospective life-event studies. In Dohrenwend, B. S., & Dohrenwend, B. P. (Eds.), *Stressful life events: Their nature and effects.* New York: Wiley, 1974.

Kagan, A. R., & Levi, L. Health and environment—psychosocial stimuli: A review. *Social Science and Medicine,* 1974, *8,* 225–241.

Kellman, S. G. Stressful life events and illness: A research area in need of development. In Dohrenwend, B. S., & Dohrenwend, B. P. (Eds.), *Stressful life events: Their nature and effects.* New York: Wiley, 1974.

Klerman, G. L., & Izen, J. E. The effects of grief and bereavement on physical health and general well-being. In Reichsman, F. (Ed.), *Advances in psychosomatic medicine: Epidemiologic studies in psychosomatic medicine.* Basel, Switzerland: S. Karger, 1974.

Langner, T. S., & Michael, S. T. *Life stress and mental health: The midtown Manhattan study* (Vol. 2, Thomas A. C. Rennie Series in Social Psychiatry). London: Collier-Macmillan, 1963.

Lazarus, R. S. Psychological stress and coping in adaptation and illness. *International Journal of Psychiatry in Medicine,* 1974, *5*(4), 321–333.

Markush, R. E., & Favero, R. V. Epidemiologic assessment of stressful life events, depressed mood, and psychophysiological symptoms—A preliminary report. In Dohrenwend, B. S., & Dohrenwend, B. P. (Eds.), *Stressful life events: Their nature and effects.* New York: Wiley, 1974.

McBride, A. B. *A Married Feminist.* New York: Harper & Row, 1976.

Mechanic, D. Discussion of research programs on relations between stressful life events and episodes of physical illness. In Dohrenwend, B. S., & Dohrenwend, B. P. (Eds.), *Stressful life events: Their nature and effects.* New York: Wiley, 1974.

Money, J., & Ehrhardt, A. *Man and woman, boy and girl.* New York: New American Library, 1974.

Myers, J. K., Lindenthal, J. J., & Pepper, M. P. Social class, life events, and psychiatric symptoms: A longitudinal study. In Dohrenwend, B. S., & Dohrenwend, B. P. (Eds.), *Stressful life events: Their nature and effects.* New York: Wiley, 1974.

Nelson, P. D. Comment. In Gunderson, E. K. E., & Rahe, R. H., *Life stress and illness.* Springfield, Ill.: Charles C Thomas, 1974.

Nuckolls, C., Cassell, J., & Kaplan, B. Psychosocial assets, life change and the prognosis of pregnancy. *American Journal of Epidemiology,* 1972, *95,* 431–441.

Paykel, E. S. Life stress and psychiatric disorders: Applications of the clinical approach. In Dohrenwend, B. S., & Dohrenwend, B. P. (Eds.), *Stressful life events: Their nature and effects.* New York: Wiley, 1974.

Paykel, E. S. Recent life events and clinical depression. In Gunderson, E. K. E., & Rahe, R. H., *Life stress and illness.* Springfield, Ill.: Charles C Thomas, 1974b.

Paykel, E. S., Prusoff, B. A., & Uhlenhuth, E. H. Scaling of life events. *Archives of General Psychiatry,* 1971, *25,* 340–347.

Pearlin, L. Sex roles and depression. In Datan, N., & Ginsberg, L. (Eds.), *Life-span developmental psychology: Normative life crises.* New York: Academic Press, 1975a.

Pearlin, L. The structure of coping. Unpublished manuscript, 1975. (b)

Pearlin, L., & Johnson, J. Marital status, life-strains and depression. Unpublished manuscript, 1975.

Rabkin, J. G., & Struening, E. L. Life events, stress, and illness. *Science,* 1976, *194,* 1013–1020.

Radloff, L. Sex differences in depression: The effects of occupation and marital status. *Sex Roles: A Journal of Research,* 1975, *1*(3), 249–266.

Radloff, L. Sex differences in mental health: The effects of marital and occupational status. Draft of text for presentation at APHA, New Orleans, 1974.

Rahe, R. H. The pathway between subjects' recent life changes and their near-future illness reports: Representative results and methodological issues. In Dohrenwend, B. S., & Dohrenwend, B. P. (Eds.), *Stressful life events: Their nature and effects.* New York: Wiley, 1974.

Rosenberg, E. J.,& Dohrenwend, B. S. Effects of experience and ethnicity on ratings of life events as stressors. *Journal of Health and Social Behavior,* 1975, *16*(1), 127–129.

Seidenberg, R. *Corporate wives— Corporate casualties?* Garden City, New York: Anchor Press/Doubleday, 1975.

Thurlow, H. J. Illness in relation to life situation and sick-role tendency. *Journal of Psychosomatic Research,* 1971, *15,* 73–88.

Uhlenhuth, E. H., Lipman, R. S., Balter, M. B., & Stern, M. Symptom intensity and life stress in the city. *Archives of General Psychiatry,* 1974, *31,* 759–764.

Wilkins, W. L. Social stress and illness in industrial society. In Gunderson, E. K. E., & Rahe, R. H. *Life Stress and Illness. Springfield, Ill.: Charles C Thomas, 1974.*

Winters, E. E. (Ed.) *The Collected Papers of Adolph Meyer* (Vol. 3, *Medical Teaching*). Baltimore: The Johns Hopkins Press, 1951.

Chapter 7

TAILORING EVALUATION TO MEASURE THE ACCOUNTABILITY OF MENTAL HEALTH SERVICES TO WOMEN

Thomas J. Kiresuk
Susan K. Schultz
James W. Baxter

The women's movement has been and continues to be a social catalyst of great power. It has been primarily responsible for the increasing awareness of sexism, the reassessment of values, the challenge to social conventions, and the thrust to legislate political equality for women. Within the behavioral sciences and the mental health service industry, this is a time for considering women's issues. In the behavioral sciences, for example, the effects of sexism on theories and research paradigms are being explored. The influence of sex-role stereotyping on personality development and interpersonal behavior is being examined. Under study, too, are the effects of the women's liberation movement on family and other social groups. The helping professions are examining their treatment of women, looking at both rationale and results. Also, consumer activism and the public press for accountability in general have been increasing. With this growing emphasis on accountability and attention to women, mental health service providers, evaluators, and policymakers are beginning to address the special concerns that women may have in using mental health services.

This chapter considers some special concerns that women may have as users of such services, two general approaches to measuring accountability, a specific evaluation methodology, and organizational readiness to implement accountability activities. These discussion topics may seem to be discrete and perhaps unrelated, but each is important in achieving accountability in mental health services to women. An elaboration of women's special concerns serves to focus evaluation questions. A consideration of

ISBN 0-12-310850-0

client- and program-specific approaches to accountability indicates general ways evaluation questions can be answered. Description of a specific evaluation methodology demonstrates one way that service information can be documented to measure accountability at both the client and programmatic level. Finally, discussion of planned organizational change and innovations emphasizes both the organizational context of most accountability activities and the fact that specific evaluation methodologies may be innovations requiring planned implementation. Realizing accountability of services to women will necessarily involve each of these elements. While this chapter focuses on the subgroup of women receiving psychotherapy, the ideas presented here are relevant to other mental health services.

SPECIAL CONCERNS OF WOMEN

The concerns noted here are raised largely in the psychotherapy and feminist literature and may be those of a subgroup of women who can articulate issues and in doing so be advocates for themselves. Other subgroups of women and of the general population of mental health service recipients may not be able to do these things. Thus while one aspect of accountability is reacting to concerns such as those expressed here, another is considering concerns that may not be voiced so loudly and clearly.

Some special concerns that the constituency of women may have are related to the possibility that treatment will be biased and directed toward conformity and adjustment to sex-role stereotypes. Recent research on sex-role stereotyping among mental health clinicians is of relevance in considering this issue. Women may also be concerned about whether to seek traditional or alternative feminist forms of treatment. The psychotherapy literature contains descriptions of some emergent feminist approaches to treating women. For the individual woman, two issues that may emerge are the translation of generic concerns into personally relevant ones and the assessment of individual readiness for treatment.

Stimulating and measuring accountability to women using mental health services necessitates generating information regarding these special concerns, and tailoring evaluation to address them. It is important, then, to ascertain the pervasiveness of sex-role stereotyping among clinicians and the impact of such bias on treatment. It is also important to further explore the efficacy of both traditional and alternative feminist forms of treatment. Efforts to individualize treatment will also increase the accountability of mental health services to women.

Treatment Bias

Service providers may have biases that are rooted in sex-role stereotypes and that may affect both the treatment process of and outcome expectations for women. Some research suggests that clinical service providers, both men and women, may judge the characteristics of mentally healthy males and females differently, typically in a manner consonant with sex-role stereotypes (Aslin, 1974; Broverman, Broverman, Clarkson, Rosenkrantz, and Vogel, 1970; Fabrikant, 1974). In these studies, clinicians are usually asked to characterize males and females in general. It is then inferred that these characterizations are in operation during treatment. Observation of the treatment process, which would be the methodology most appropriate for detecting treatment bias, has not been reported. It is important to acknowledge that, although references are made to a population of therapists in general, this group is no more uniform than the clients they serve (Kiesler, 1966).

The widely cited study by Broverman *et al.* (1970), finds the mentally healthy female to be characterized by clinicians as more submissive, less independent, more passive, more easily influenced, more excitable in a minor crisis, more emotional, less logical, less self-confident, more conceited about appearance, and more subjective than her male counterpart: a questionable picture of mental health for anyone. The mentally healthy male and the sex-unspecified adult were characterized as manifesting traits judged to be more socially desirable by a sample of nonclinical subjects. Healthy males and sex-unspecified adults were seen as generally more competitive, worldly, direct, skilled in business, adventurous, ambitious, and as having an easier time making decisions than healthy females.

Some persons in the mental health field have taken this research as evidence of a double standard of mental health. Stricker (1977), however, emphasizes that this conclusion may be questionable in light of the Broverman *et al.* (1970) methodology and moreover that the generalizability of inferences from such analogue data to the treatment situation has not been tested. Stricker cites a recent study by Maxfield (1976) of sex-role stereotyping among members of the American Psychological Association's Division of Psychotherapy. This study, which obtained a 25% response rate among the approximately 1000 experienced therapists sampled, contradicts the conclusions of Broverman *et al.* (1970). Maxfield (1976) and Stricker (1977) concur that no evidence exists to suggest an overall bias against women among clinicians.

The pervasiveness of sex-role stereotyping among clinicians and the effect of such stereotypic views on the treatment process are issues that require further investigation. If service providers do perceive the mental health of males and females differently, then different treatment expectations based on sex of the client are possible, as are different perceptions of what constitutes successful treatment. Treatment that is biased by sex-role stereotypes may encourage a woman's adjustment to that stereotypic role and may implicitly or explicitly foster, for example, dependence rather than independence, passivity rather than assertiveness, marriage rather than another lifestyle, or the role of homemaker rather than a career outside the home.

The Task Force on Sex Bias and Sex-Role Stereotyping in Psychotherapeutic Practice (Brodsky, Holroyd, Payton, Rubinstein, Rosenkrantz, Sherman, & Zell, 1975) suggests that although little information exists, biased treatment may be manifested in different ways for women with particular characteristics. For example, certain prejudices may exist regarding low-income women. Similarly, women who are members of racial minorities or who are lesbians may experience biased treatment related to membership in one of those subgroups. For example, all lesbians, regardless of accompanying clinical features, may be judged by some to be emotionally disturbed and may be encouraged to establish a "good" heterosexual relationship as a solution to their "problem," without this value judgment being made explicit or the preferences of the client being fully considered.

There are likely to be different treatment expectations not based on biased judgment for subgroups of women (and men) who have particular characteristics. It is unrealistic to expect similar outcomes for all persons who are provided mental health services. A women experiencing her first serious depression in the context of a life crisis begins treatment in a different state and with a different treatment outcome expectation than a woman with a history of recurrent, severe psychotic depressions. Depending on other resources and liabilities—physical, social, economic, and personal—the former may be judged as having a good service outcome if she experiences less depression, feels hopeful about her life, and resumes occupational activities with enthusiasm. The latter may be judged as having a good outcome if her delusions recede and she is able to function in a day treatment program. In light of the potential for treatment bias, women using mental health services may be concerned about whether the gender of the service provider will make a difference in their treatment. Orlinsky and Howard (1976) reanalyzed questionnaire data collected from 118 women who received dynamically-oriented individual outpatient psychotherapy at an urban mental health clinic. The women provided multifaceted descriptions of their therapy session experiences. The range of session reports per woman was 5 to 66. From these reports, factor analysis produced a set of dimensions that, when analyzed as a function of the therapist's gender, suggests that single women and depressed women experience greater support and satisfaction in treatment with a female therapist. The effect of the therapist's gender on a woman's therapy needs to be studied further in other clinical samples and settings, as does relationship between gender of the therapist and a woman's therapy outcome.

Another related concern for women using mental health services may be the experience of sexual attraction and the potential for sexual intimacy between therapist and client, which has been reported in the case of a male therapist and female client. According to the Task Force on Sex Bias and Sex-Role Stereotyping in Psychotherapeutic Practice (Brodsky *et al.*, 1975), this situation both exploits the stereotypic feminine qualities of the woman client and exerts the dominant power of the therapist. The Task Force also reports that the psychotherapeutic literature has not documented any positive effects of sexual intimacy between a therapist and client, and anecdotal testimony has suggested this practice may be greatly destructive to the woman. There is little doubt that sexual intimacy between therapist and client constitutes exploitation and unethical conduct on the part of the therapist.

Traditional or Alternative Treatment?

Women may be concerned about whether to accept traditional dynamic therapy or to seek alternative feminist forms of treatment. Traditional dynamic therapy for women includes more than one therapeutic style, theory, and strategy. However, the various styles and strategies of traditional therapy have been discussed by some as rooted in personality theory that is biased and inadequately descriptive of women (Carlson, 1972; Doherty, 1973). Traditional therapy has been criticized for typically stressing internal and intrapsychic causes of women's problems rather than external and environmental causes. Traditional therapy has also been criticized for seeking individual solutions to women's problems and encouraging adjustment to the status quo (Rawlings & Carter, 1977).

Chesler (1972) has argued that traditional psychotherapy typically devalues women and fosters traditional sex-roles. She has concluded that women therapy clients should be treated only by female clinicians who are feminists. Her critique of traditional psychotherapy is that it isolates women from each other and typically places the female client in an all too familiar and stereotypic position of submission to a powerful male—in this instance, the therapist.

Feminist therapy has evolved in reaction to the perceived inadequacies of traditional therapy for women. Mander and Rush (1974) have described feminist therapy as a synthesis of traditional therapies and developments in the women's movement.

From the feminist perspective, many personal problems women experience are the result of a social, cultural, and political environment that is oppressive to women. In a phrase, the "personal is political." While feminists politicize women's problems, traditional mental health treatment of women has been observed to ignore the political (Chesler, 1972; Kirsh, 1974).

Value assumptions and strategies of emergent nonsexist and feminist therapies have been articulated (Feminist Counseling Collective, 1975; Sprei-Ott, 1976; Thomas, 1977). Rawlings and Carter (1977) have described nonsexist therapy as involving a therapist aware of his or her own values, prescribing no sex-role behaviors, accepting sex-role reversals, and considering marriage as no better a treatment outcome for females than males. A nonsexist therapist would also expect males and females to similarly achieve autonomy, assertiveness, expressiveness, and tenderness, and finally, would reject behavioral theories based on anatomical differences. Rawlings and Carter have characterized feminist therapy as sharing the assumptions of nonsexist therapy and also assuming that women's inferior status is related to their having less political and economic power than men, attributing women's pathology primarily to social and external rather than personal and internal sources, and opposing personal adjustment to social conditions. A feminist therapist would also assert that women must be economically and psychologically autonomous, and advocate the eradication of major differences between "appropriate" sex-role behaviors for men and women.

Klein (1976) considers feminist concepts of therapy outcome for women and how they may differ from traditional concepts. She has suggested that judgment of a favorable outcome from a traditional perspective may assume that what is good for society must be good for the individual, while judgment of a favorable outcome from a feminist perspective may assume the converse, that what is good for the woman may not always be good for society. The feminist perspective may even attribute a woman's mental illness to social conditions rather than to other causes. While the traditional concept of outcome may emphasize adjustment to role expectations, the feminist concept may emphasize changing those roles or role expectations. Klein also notes that a traditionally positive outcome of psychotherapy has been a client's ability to demonstrate more warmth, expressiveness, and nurturance in relationships. However, from a feminist perspective, this treatment outcome for a woman may move her even closer to stereotypic female role behavior and farther from behavior unbounded by that stereotype.

With politicizing of personal problems in mind, feminists have evolved alternatives to traditional psychotherapy for women. These include consciousness-raising (CR) groups, self-help groups, assertiveness training, and feminist bibliotherapy. CR groups (Brodsky [1977]; Kravetz [1976]), unlike most therapy groups, assume that the social environment rather than intrapsychic forces are the root of many women's problems and thus seek to bring women together to share experiences and to serve as role models for each other. CR groups tend to be more topic-oriented than individual-oriented, generally placing problems women face in a social and political context. Glaser (1976) has described self-help groups for women as a complement to CR group experiences.

Assertiveness training for women has been described as an alternative clinical technique for treating women experiencing a range of problems (Jakubowski, 1977). Among problems that have been treated in part by assertiveness training are neurotic depression, child abuse, chemical dependency, psychosomatic problems, and problems related to jobs, dating, and couple communication. Feminist bibliotherapy has also been discussed as an alternative treatment for women (Sanders & Stewart, 1977). This typically involves providing the woman with reading material geared to help her identify external determinants of her problems and pain, and to initiate her examination of her own socialization. It is noteworthy that in general, mental health services are not politicized. Thus, the arguments regarding politicizing personal problems may be applicable to consumer constituencies other than women.

Individualized Treatment

The woman using mental health services may be concerned about the translation of general information and concerns regarding women into the context of personally relevant events. The process of translation is a familiar one. For example, a woman may conclude accurately that while her depression is similar to that of others, it is also somewhat different. Her role conflicts may be nothing new but they are hers, made unique by her genetic and environmental history, her past life experiences and learning, and her emotional and social resources. This woman may ask, "In guiding me toward growth and health, how will this particular treatment take into account what is known about women in general and what is known about me personally?" She may be concerned that the person providing her treatment be informed of and accommodate her unique characteristics, capabilities, needs, and aspirations. She must incorporate consumer information regarding therapist, treatment, and setting and her own knowledge of self into her decision-making regarding mental health services.

One woman may demand evidence that her therapist hold to an androgynous model of mental health while another woman may be fearful that something called "feminism" will be foisted upon her. Although they may differ in orientation women share the concern that mental health services and service providers be responsive to them as individuals. Elements of the concern include: an explicit consideration of values, articulation of treatment goals and criteria for successful outcome, and importantly, a tailoring of treatment to changes a woman is ready to make.

A woman's readiness for treatment is an issue, particularly in the context of a diverse constituency of women, therapists, and treatments. Some aspects of therapy, feminist or otherwise, may be inappropriate for a particular woman, in a particular place, at a particular time. The assessment of each woman's readiness for treatment is one way to tailor therapy to that woman. Such assessment may serve to focus treatment on the individual woman, who may share special concerns with other women but who may also embody concerns and characteristics unique to her.

ADDRESSING CONCERNS OF WOMEN

The potential for treatment bias, the choice between traditional and alternative forms of treatment, and the individualization of treatment have been noted as special concerns women may have in using mental health services. These special concerns need to be addressed in measuring the accountability of services to women.

Accountability is a word heard with increasing frequency in mental health service settings. In this context, accountability means the ability to justify to funding sources, regulatory agencies, and consumers what services are offered, how they are provided, and how much they cost. Speaking to a medical audience, Densen (1973) simply defines accountability as the responsibility of reporting the operation and effectiveness of health care programs.

Accountability activities pursue the exposition of motivational structures and rationales, operational facts, and values that underpin service provision. Making these underpinnings of service provision explicit is a central purpose of accountability endeavors. To the extent that psychotherapy and other mental health services are not and cannot be free of value systems, it is the responsibility of those providing the services to make their values as well as other service underpinnings and agenda items open to scrutiny, and in so doing, to become accountable to their constituencies, one being women.

Quality assurance and program evaluation represent the primary categorical approaches to measuring and ensuring accountability (Woy, Lund, & Attkisson, 1978). In quality assurance, the level of analysis is generally client-specific; typically, individual treatment records are audited to review the quality of care. In program evaluation, the level of analysis is generally program-specific and often involves examination of aggregate program data to assess program effectiveness. Both approaches could be tailored to address special concerns of women; each is important in decision-making directed at improving services and programs for women.

Quality assurance activities have been extensively legislated during the past ten years. They are required in inpatient health settings, including psychiatric facilities for medicare and medicaid reimbursement. The Joint Commission on Accreditation of Hospitals (JCAH) and Public Law 92–63, which authorizes Professional Standards Review Organizations (PSROs), both mandate quality assurance measures in such settings. PSRO review is currently optional in outpatient settings. However, the Community Mental Health Center amendments of 1975, found in Title III of Public Law 94–63, require that Community Mental Health Centers (CMHCs) with federal funding establish quality assurance activities. These amendments also require that each federally-funded CMHC perform ongoing evaluation of its programs and services.

Quality Assurance of Services to Women

Quality assurance of mental health services that women receive is an issue that cuts across traditional and alternative forms of treatment. Historically, quality assurance has tried to define and maintain professional and administrative standards with specific objectives to assure that individual clients receive appropriate care, identify and correct service provision deficiencies or errors, and control cost of care by preventing overutilization and by giving instruction in efficient provision of needed services. Methodologies for assessing quality of care have emphasized peer review. This audit of service records by professional peers typically involves a comparison of service provided a particular client with professionally developed standards or criteria of appropriate and adequate service. Assessments may be concurrent or retrospective in nature. Concurrent reviews consider the level of service provision and assess appropriate and economical provision of continued service. Retrospective reviews study quality of care variables and monitor service to derive profiles or patterns of care (Woy *et al.*, 1978).

Quality reviews require that standards of care be defined and that actual practice be evaluated in light of those standards. The focal question in audit is how can the quality of care be improved? The Foundation for

Health Care Evaluation (1977) has outlined twelve steps necessary for an effective audit of care. The audit process requires that clinicians meet to consider quality of care, what should be documented in the treatment record, and specifically to act upon the following steps.

1. Select a topic or problem to audit, such as a psychiatric diagnosis, a particular problem, or a special concern such as treatment bias.
2. Establish audit criteria including elements of care, standards, exceptions, and instructions for retrieving the needed data from treatment records. Criteria are usually given a 100% or 0% standard, which means that a specific criterion is to be followed always or never. Three audit criteria with a 100% standard that might be found in an outpatient mental health clinic quality review are (*a*) consumer information is provided, (*b*) readiness for treatment is evaluated and recorded by the second visit, and (*c*) treatment goals are recorded by the third visit.
3. Examine the criteria to assure that they are relevant, understandable, measurable, behavioral, and achievable.
4. Compare the criteria to actual practice as documented in the clinical records.
5. Identify practices which vary from the criteria.
6. Determine whether each variation from the criteria is justified or represents a care problem.
7. Evaluate the factors relating to the problem in care.
8. Consider and assess the alternatives for correcting the problem.
9. Select and initiate an action plan to correct the problem.
10. After implementation, evaluate the efficacy of the plan to correct the problem. Based on this evaluation continue the plan or initiate another.
11. Report the results of the corrective action to appropriate parties such as clinicians, administrators, and consumers.
12. Reassess the problem at a predetermined future date to determine the long-term effectiveness of the corrective plan.

The quality assurance process and the audit steps associated with traditional therapies are the same for the alternative therapies. Relevant points of view require conversion into measurable criteria in order to be used in audit and accountability reviews. The review process must be carried out faithfully and the outcomes assessed fairly.

Questions related to bias are difficult to evaluate, particularly since standards of mental health care for women are sketchy or nonexistent. Quality review presumes the existence of adequate care criteria or standards against which to compare actual treatment. While consensual standards for women's mental health care are not now available, the beginnings of such standards are, in the form of increasing knowledge regarding psychology of women and women's mental health and articulation of feminist concerns. Responsible clinicians may begin to incorporate this knowledge into their reviews of quality of care for women. This incorporation will necessitate grappling with the definition of bias and how to discern from treatment records evidence of such bias. Quality reviews will ideally allow peer groups of clinicians to interact on the special concerns of women receiving treatment, to enhance their consciousness regarding treatment of women, and in practice to define and evolve improved care for women.

Quality assurance reviews have special relevance to subgroups of women who are not capable of self-advocacy. Although many women using mental health services have the ability to advocate on their own behalf and have great potential for personal growth and change, others do not. For some women using mental health services, the pursuit of consumer information, therapist-client value explication, and the ability to articulate quality of care issues are not possible. Some women in treatment are profoundly retarded, some are mute in mental illness, others are actively delusional, and others are in emotional crisis. For these women, protection and audit of their mental health care must come from review by mental health professional peers, trained technicians or consumer advocates.

Evaluation of Programs Serving Women

The evaluation of mental health services to women is important in addressing questions of effective and efficient programming for women. Both traditional and alternative programs for women must be evaluated to enhance their operation and to judge their worth. Program evaluation activities have generally addressed questions of program effort, outcome, efficiency, and impact with specific objectives to maintain high levels of program effort devoted to attaining program goals, identify and maintain programs that are cost-efficient when considering their outcomes, and acquire sensitivity to the intended and unintended impact of program effort on a particular community or constituency. Figure 7.1 identifies four types of evaluation and their subcomponents, which reflect that evaluation may encompass a wide range of activities. Evaluation methodologies range from ex post facto analysis to experimental design and often focus on comparison of program performance to program goals. Evaluation may be summative or formative in nature (Scriven, 1972). Summative evaluation occurs once after the conclusion of the program. Results have generally been used to judge the ultimate value of a program and to decide whether

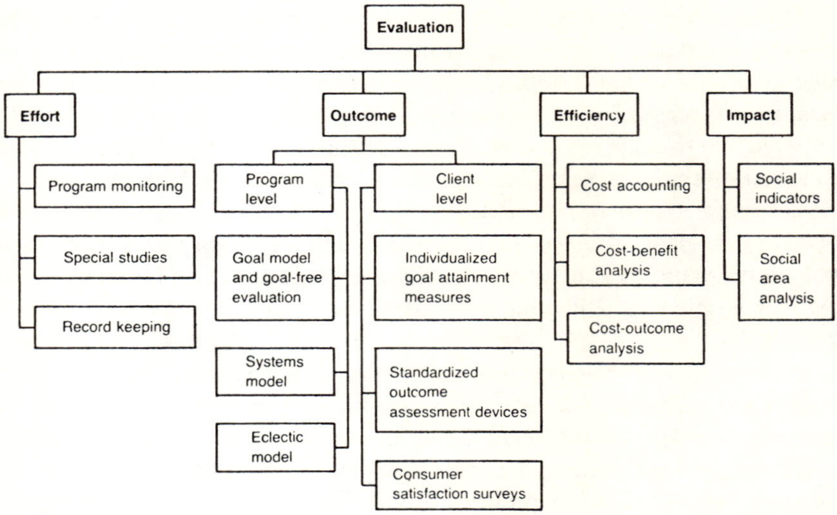

FIGURE 7.1 Four major types of evaluation and their subcomponents. [Reproduced by permission of the publisher from Wayne Anderson, Bernard J. Frieden, and Michael Murphy, eds., *Managing Human Services* (Washington, D.C.: International City Management Association, 1977), p. 288.]

its implementation elsewhere is warranted. Formative evaluation occurs periodically during the course of a program and results have generally been used as feedback to improve organizational operations and service provision.

Goal-oriented evaluations allow a program to be self-correcting by producing performance information relevant to program goals for substantive feedback to improve performance and better meet goals. Walker and Baxter (1972) have demonstrated that giving mental health service providers feedback may enhance the attainment of client goals.

Evaluation can also provide information that addresses issues beyond the scope of an individual program. In this context it may be useful to aggregate evaluative information across programs to consider questions of relevance to the general constituency of women or to a particular subgroup. Examination of goals across programs for women could reveal whether programming is addressing special concerns of women. For example, programs that do not consider the effects of sexism in the treatment of women—either through staff consciousness-raising goals or as evidenced through the goals of services provided—may be inadequately responding to concerns of many women. Examination of summative evaluations across kinds of services for women could suggest successful areas of programming and program development for women. Consideration of goals and evaluations of programs serving women across the nation could highlight regions that are more or less responsive to women's concerns. With this information, strategies to educate regions regarding special concerns of women and to promote responsiveness to these concerns could be formulated by organizations of clinical professionals or other advocacy groups.

The efficacy of mental health services and programs in alleviating problems women experience is an important evaluation question. In the long run, however, evaluation must also consider the impact that programming has on the constituency of women and its subgroups. A point of view stressed by many is that the evaluation of programming for women should measure whether or not such programs prevent problems. Can mental health programming for women be shown to have a significant impact on problem rates among women? The design and measurement problems in this area are most challenging, but the women and the public in general will require some such evidence if the costs of maintaining and developing special programs are to be supported.

MEASURING ACCOUNTABILITY TO WOMEN

Measuring the accountability of mental health services to women by doing either quality assurance audits or program evaluation requires that treatment records be kept and that instances of care be documented. More than one way to record and document treatment has been proposed and implemented (Ellis & Wilson, 1973; Kiresuk & Sherman, 1968; Weed, 1969). Goal Attainment Scaling (GAS) is presented here as a record-keeping and evaluation methodology that could be helpful to women's services and programs interested in developing accountability systems. Its discussion here illustrates one approach to measuring accountability.

The method involves the recording of client-specific information on a Goal Attainment Follow-Up Guide, which is a paper grid designed to document treatment goals and outcome levels. The method requires that on the follow-up guide, individualized treatment goals be articulated, that expected and possible goal outcome levels be specified, that actual outcome levels be recorded, and that a score be computed across goal areas to summarize individual goal attainment. (See appendix for a detailed description of the GAS background and methodology.)

A measurement device such as GAS serves as an important bridge between the recognition of women's special concerns in using mental health services and the realization of accountability to that constituency. It records the purposes of treatment, provides an index of individual progress, and offers evidence of therapeutic intent and outcome. This kind of evidence is essential to answering questions on accountability. The information on a follow-up guide could be used to assess the quality of individual care while information from many guides could be aggregated to answer program evaluation questions. What follows is a brief description of how GAS might be used for quality assurance audit and program evaluation.

USING GOAL ATTAINMENT SCALING IN EVALUATION AND AUDIT

GAS is a tool that has been used variously in the evaluation of programs. When GAS has been used to set service goals with clients, then goal attainment scores have been organized to reflect program effectiveness. In the original application of GAS, the basic purpose was to compare the effectiveness of different treatment modes. This involved three basic steps: (*a*) constructing a follow-up guide for the client during the intake process, (*b*) random assignment to a treatment mode, and (*c*) follow-up at a predetermined time interval.

GAS can be used to explore and compare the efficacy of new treatments for women. For example, using GAS as the outcome measure, the efficacy of CR group experience, assertiveness training, individual feminist therapy, and traditional psychotherapy could be compared. Designs of evaluation involving more than one treatment have accommodated both ethics of treatment assignment and the judgment that a client should experience more than one of the treatments.

Use of GAS in this way might suggest which treatment modes are more or less successful in dealing with specific problem and goal areas. For example, within the context of a hypothetical program, a formative evaluation might indicate that for women experiencing certain problems, outcomes are better among those assigned to assertiveness training than among those assigned to CR groups or individual psychotherapy. The programmatic response to this evaluation might be the routine assignment of women experiencing those problems to assertiveness training unless there are individual and specific reasons not to do so.

The Goal Attainment Follow-Up Guide could be one element of a woman's mental health treatment record used in a concurrent review of care. The Hennepin County Mental Health Service outpatient department in Minneapolis, Minnesota, has used an audit form to rate the follow-up guides of clients for general aspects of quality, such as to determine whether scales are relevant and realistic, or in need of modification. An audit form reflecting these issues is represented in Figure 7.2.

Date: *July 15, 1973* Current Report Period: *June 1, 1973* to *June 30, 1973* Prepared by: *Dreyer*

ITEM NUMBER	RESPONSE OPTION	CURRENT MONTH NUMBER SCALES	CURRENT MONTH PERCENT	LAST MONTH NUMBER SCALES	LAST MONTH PERCENT	CUMULATIVE TOTAL NUMBER SCALES	CUMULATIVE TOTAL PERCENT
1. Are the scales relevant?	YES	7	70	76	92	541	91
	NO	3	30	7	8	34	6
	BLANK	0	0	0	0	3	3
	TOTAL	10	100%	83	100%	578	100%
2. Are the scales realistic?	1—VERY PESSIMISTIC	0	0	0	0	2	.4
	2—PESSIMISTIC	0	0	7	9	34	7
	3—RIGHT ON	6	86	53	70	380	78
	4—OPTIMISTIC	0	0	9	12	47	9
	5—VERY OPTIMISTIC	1	14	7	9	14	3
	BLANK	0	0	0	0	13	2.6
	TOTAL	7	100%	76	100%	490	100%
3. Would you modify scale weights	YES	0	0	2	3	13	3
	NO	7	100	70	92	437	89
	BLANK	0	0	4	5	40	8
	TOTAL	7	100%	76	100%	490	100%
4. Would you modify scale levels?	YES	1	14	7	9	35	. 7
	NO	6	86	66	87	437	89
	BLANK	0	0	3	4	18	4
	TOTAL	7	100%	76	100%	490	100%
5. Would you add any scales?	YES	0	0	8	28	36	20
	NO	7	100	20	69	139	78
	BLANK	0	0	1	3	4	2
	TOTAL	7	100%	29	100%	179	100%

FIGURE 7.2. Hennepin County Mental Health Service, outpatient department; Minneapolis, Minnesota: Intake goal attainment guide assessment rating report.

Follow-up guides could be part of an audit for special concerns of women using mental health services. In auditing for a concern such as treatment bias, the information from follow-up guides would likely need to be supplemented with information from other treatment records. What from the content of scales on a guide alone might appear to be evidence of treatment toward sex-role conformity may in fact reflect appropriate setting of goals for that woman at that time in light of other information. Conversely, a follow-up guide constructed to reflect a woman's liberation, containing content related to independent living, higher education, and consciousness raising, may in the context of more information be premature, reflecting treatment aiming toward such behaviors without the woman herself being ready for it.

Concurrent audit using GAS might be usefully incorporated into a clinical case conference. This would allow the assessment of guide quality by clinical peers, a review process which quickly becomes routine, and discussion among clinicians of more difficult issues such as bias. Audit for the quality of guide construction is a task that can be appropriately assumed by a trained clerical worker rather than clinician. At this time, however, the criteria for audit of treatment bias are not clear enough.

Retrospective review of follow-up guides could involve the aggregation of goal content and goal attainment scores for women generally, or for subgroups of women, to derive profiles and patterns of care. For example, it would be possible to derive patterns of care for women going through divorce, in terms of the problems they dealt with as represented by scale headings, and the accuracy of service outcome predictions as represented by goal attainment scores. The same could be done for single parents, rape victims, or women with specific diagnoses. A pattern of service for women going through divorce that does not reflect expected referrals to legal resources may suggest an area of care that is deficient. Similarly, a pattern of service for rape victims in which goals considering anger are expected but found to be rare may warrant a closer look at both the client population and the provision of care.

Using goal attainment follow-up guides, quality review, and evaluation research regarding treatment goals and outcomes across a large sample of women and clinicians could provide information useful in better tailoring mental health services for women. Analysis of specific clinical interventions and modes of treatment in the context of types of clients, problems, goals, and outcomes may also produce useful information. Although some findings will no doubt be expected, it is likely that there will be surprises, with new and unexpected discoveries regarding the treatment of women emerging.

Organizational Readiness to Implement Accountability Activities

For programs that wish to implement GAS or other accountability mechanisms, assessment of the organization's readiness to adopt an innovation may guide their strategies of implementation. Factors affecting the successful adoption of an innovation and planned organizational change have been considered by many theorists (Glaser, 1973; Havelock & Lingwood, 1973). Davis (1971) has developed the A VICTORY model which describes eight determinants of organizational change. Figure 7.3 represents the A VICTORY dimensions of organization change and names the categories within those dimensions that are of particular relevance to program evaluation. Based on Davis' model, the "Organizational Readiness to Accept Program Evaluation Questionnaire" has been developed (Kiresuk, Lund, Schultz, & Larsen, 1977). It has been administered to the staff of some programs to facilitate the actual implementation of accountability procedures.

A profile of organizational readiness for such implementation can be derived from the analysis of questionnaire responses by all or a representative group of a program staff. This profile reflects organizational conditions thought to promote or hamper adoption of innovation. Figure 7.4 represents the profile of one organization's climate for implementation of program evaluation procedures. Points to the left of the midscale indicate potential problems for adoption of innovation.

The profile of this example organization indicates that history of support for change and employment or personnel policies may hamper innovation adoption. To facilitate adoption, organizational meetings considering these staff perceptions and explicit administrative support and policy for change may be necessary. In addition, the Department of Social Work staff profile of this organization indicates that they do not have enough information regarding the planned changes nor do they feel much pressure to evaluate. Informational meetings or materials regarding the planned changes and the external pressures for accountability may be simple strategies useful in encouraging these workers to be more amenable to the introduction of innovations.

This kind of readiness analysis is one way to lay the groundwork for implementation of accountability activities. Not all organizations planning such implementation will utilize this process of assessing readiness for change. What is important is that climate for change is assessed in some manner to guide implementation. Another form of questionnaire, a checklist, interviews with staff, or staff meetings might all be used to assess an

ABILITY

Category 1: Willingness and ability to commit resources to program evaluation.

Category 2: Present availability and skill level of manpower to plan and implement program evaluation. Knowledge of program evaluation methods by those concerned.

VALUES

Category 3: Attitudes and beliefs of those involved toward accepting program evaluation.

Category 4: Organization's history of change, and history of support for change.

Category 5: Characteristics of staff or administrators thought to bear on acceptance of program evaluation (other than attitudes or skill level).

Category 6: Work relations; supervisory relations; interpersonal relations.

Category 7: Employment or personnel policies of the organization (i.e., of the employer).

INFORMATION

Category 8: Availability of information bearing on program's present functioning. Availability and use of procedures and channels for recording and communicating program information.

CIRCUMSTANCES

Category 9: Aspects of the program relating to procedures, job duties, job requirements, and job expectations.

Category 10: Quality of the relationship between the program and those it serves and those it works with.

TIMING

Category 11: Timing of program evaluation to coincide or coordinate with other program or organizational activities.

OBLIGATION

Category 12: Felt need to "do something," to take action. Pressure to evaluate. Awareness of present danger to or health of program.

RESISTANCE

Category 13: Expected or feared negative consequences of program evaluation. Frontstage or backstage fears of loss resulting from adoption of program evaluation.

YIELD

Category 14: Expected or hoped for positive consequences of program evaluation. Payoff or rewards thought to result from adopting program evaluation.

FIGURE 7.3. A VICTORY dimensions for organization assessment. [Reprinted from *Evaluation,* Volume 4, 1977 by permission of copyright holder Minneapolis Medical Research Foundation, Inc.]

organization's readiness and make the implementation process more efficient and successful.

SUMMARY

Tailoring evaluation to measure the accountability of mental health services to women will necessarily involve at least four areas of consideration or activity: (*a*) considering special concerns that women may have in using such services; (*b*) approaching questions of accountability at both the client and program level of analysis; (*c*) selecting an evaluation methodol-

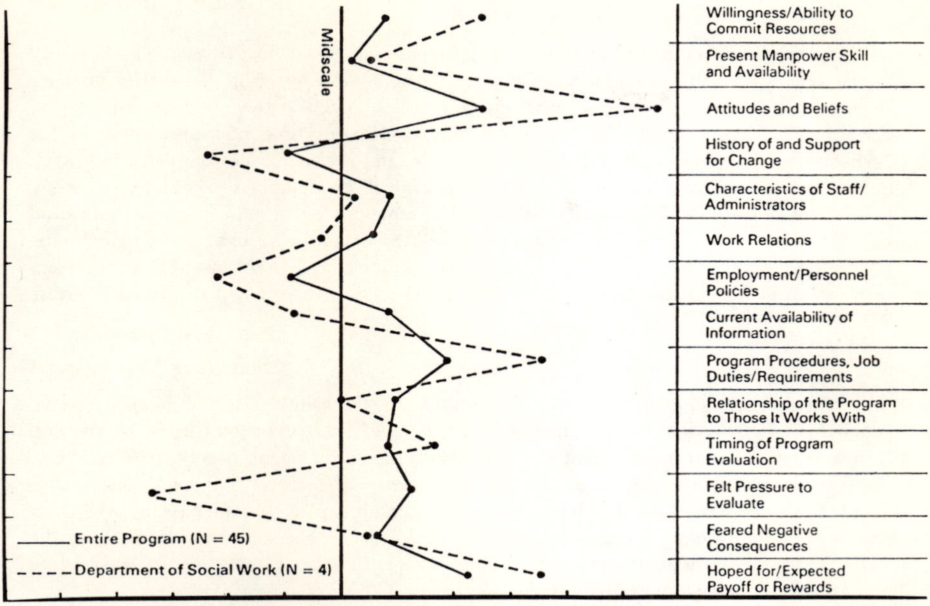

FIGURE 7.4. Sample organization readiness profiles. [Reprinted from *Evaluation,* Volume 4, 1977 by permission of copyright holder Minneapolis Medical Research Foundation, Inc.]

ogy that can address special concerns at the client and program level; and (*d*) planning the implementation of accountability activities with the specific organizational environment and its readiness for change in mind. Thus, encouraging mental health services to be accountable to women will be a multifaceted enterprise.

APPENDIX

Background and Methodology of Goal Attainment Scaling

GAS was originally applied at the Hennepin County Mental Health Service in Minneapolis in response to that program's obligation "to do program evaluation." Kiresuk and Sherman (1968) developed the method to meet accountability requirements and at the same time to provide for the unique characteristics of the treatment process and the aspirations of individual clients. Their primary objective was to design a measure capable of determining mental health service effectiveness. They set no limits on content, because fixed standards of mental health could not be attributed to all service providers or applied to all clients. They assumed that service providers could predict with reasonable accuracy how service would affect client problems or goals. In designing GAS, they attempted to accommodate the values of the client, treatment staff, and the service organization. The method involves individually relevant goal areas, a weighting system among the goals, expected outcome statements, follow-up scoring of outcomes, and a score summarizing the outcomes across all of the goal areas.

Guide Construction

A key factor in the GAS methodology is preparation of the Goal Attainment Follow-up Guide, which is a grid-shaped form designating five outcome levels. This preparation involves seven steps: selecting goal areas, weighting the scales to reflect their relative importance, choosing goal attainment indicators, establishing a follow-up time interval, completing the "expected level," completing additional scale levels, and reviewing the completed follow-up guide. The process of preparing a follow-up guide will be described in terms of a young woman treated in a crisis intervention center. The same process of guide construction would be followed with any client and also has been followed in organizational and programmatic goal-setting (Kiresuk & Lund, 1977). The woman in this example is not meant to be representative of women receiving mental health services. Her follow-up guide is displayed in Figure 7.5.

Selecting Goal Areas

The first step in constructing a follow-up guide is the identification of major concerns, problem areas, or goal areas to be included on the guide. This can be done using information from a variety of sources, including the client, professional judgment, past records, relatives, or others. In this case, the therapist and woman together selected five goal areas. Once a goal area has been chosen, a word or brief phrase describing it is placed in the box at the top of a scale as a scale heading. Only scales relevant to the service endeavor are identified on the guide. The scale headings chosen for this woman were: education, suicide, manipulation, drug abuse, and dependency on crisis intervention center (CIC).

Weighting the Scales

The weighting of each scale is an optional step in the GAS process. It involves the subjective judgment of the guide constructor as to whether some of the selected goals are more important than others. The weighting process allows the reflection of the relative importance of goals on a guide. A weight may be represented by any number between 1 and 99. If one goal area is weighted, all must be weighted. Several goals may be assigned the same weight or, if all goals are considered equal in importance, no weights may be assigned. In Figure 7.5, suicide and drug abuse, both weighted 30, were considered the most important goal areas for the woman. Manipulation was next in importance, reflected by a weight of 25. Education followed with a weight of 20; dependency in CIC with a weight of 10, was considered the least urgent goal area.

Choosing Goal Attainment Indicators

The third step involves the identification of indicators that will reflect improvement or lack of it in relation to each of the designated goal areas. These indicators are defined as observable, measurable signs of progress. In some cases, the goal area is implicitly an observable, measurable behavior such as expression of anger or crying. Other goal areas, such as depression, necessitate the definition of observable and related indicators, such as continual sleeping, number of crying spells, or a score on a psychometric scale measuring depression. Indicators for the woman represented in Figure 7.5 included enrollment in high school, suicidal impulses, demands for medications, drug use, and CIC contacts.

FIGURE 7.5. Sample Goal Attainment Follow-up Guide for a crisis intervention center client. A check mark indicates level at intake. An asterisk signifies level at follow-up. [Reprinted from *Evaluation,* Special Monograph Number 1, 1973 by permission of copyright holder Minneapolis Medical Research Foundation, Inc.]

SCALE HEADINGS AND SCALE WEIGHTS

Check whether or not the scale has been mutually negotiated between patient and CIC interviewer.	Yes X No ___	Yes ___ No X	Yes ___ No X	Yes X No ___	Yes X No ___
SCALE ATTAINMENT LEVELS	SCALE 1: Education (w1=20)	SCALE 2: Suicide (w2=30)	SCALE 3: Manipulation (w3=25)	SCALE 4: Drug Abuse (w4=30)	SCALE 5: Dependency on CIC (w5=10)
a. most unfavorable treatment outcome thought likely (-2)	Patient has made no attempt to enroll in high school. ✓	Patient has committed suicide.	Patient makes rounds of community service agencies demanding medication, and refuses other forms of treatment. ✓	Patient reports addiction to "hard narcotics" (heroin, morphine).	Patient has contacted CIC by telephone or in person at least seven times since her first visit.
b. less than expected success with treatment (-1)	Patient has enrolled in high school, but at time of follow-up has dropped out.	Patient has acted on at least one suicidal impulse since her first contact with the CIC, but has not succeeded. ✓	Patient no longer visits CIC with demands for medication but continues with other community agencies and still refuses other forms of treatment.	Patient has used "hard narcotics," but is not addicted, and/or uses hallucinogens (LSD, Pot) more than four times a month. ✓	Patient has contacted CIC 5-6 times since intake. ✓
c. expected level of treatment success (0)	Patient has enrolled, and is in school at follow-up, but is attending class sporadically (misses an average of more than a third of her classes during a week).	Patient reports she has had at least four suicidal impulses since her first contact with the CIC but has not acted on any of them.	Patient no longer attempts to manipulate for drugs at community service agencies, but will not accept another form of treatment.	Patient has not used "hard narcotics" during follow-up period, and uses hallucinogens between 1-4 times a month. *	Patient has contacted CIC 3-4 times since intake.
d. more than expected success with treatment (+1)	Patient has enrolled, is in school at follow-up, and is attending classes consistently, but has no vocational goals. *	*	Patient accepts non-medication treatment at some community agency. *	Patient uses hallucinogens less than once a month.	
e. best anticipated success with treatment (+2)	Patient has enrolled, is in school at follow-up, is attending classes consistently, and has some vocational goal.	Patient reports she has had no suicidal impulses since her first contact with the CIC.	Patient accepts non-medication treatment, and by own report shows signs of improvement.	At time of follow-up, patient is not using any illegal drugs.	Patient has not contacted CIC since intake. *

Establishing Follow-up Time Interval

This fourth step involves the designation of a time frame within which it is predicted that the goals on the follow-up guide will be accomplished. The end point of this time frame is the date when the follow-up guide will be scored. The designated follow-up time interval for this woman was two months.

Completing the "Expected Level"

In selecting the expected level, an anchor point for the rest of the scale is designated. The expected level answers the question, "Realistically, what will this client be able to achieve in each goal area in a given time frame and in terms of the chosen indicators?" The woman in Figure 7.5 was expected, in a two-month period, to enroll in high school and attend sporadically, to have at least four suicidal impulses without acting on any, to not attempt to get drugs at community service agencies while refusing other treatment, to abstain from "hard narcotics" while using hallucinogens between one and four times a month, and to contact the CIC three to four times dating from intake. The reasoning behind these outcome selections went something like this. Given this woman, and considering her background, environment, abilities, liabilities and hopes, and given the capabilities of the treatment staff to treat such an individual, and considering the current state of relevant knowledge, this is what we can expect her to accomplish in two months.

Completing Additional Scale Levels

Each scale on a follow-up guide must contain five distinct possible outcome levels that are adequately detailed in writing on the guide or if blank, easily inferred from adjacent levels. The two levels on the guide immediately adjacent to the expected level— somewhat less and somewhat more treatment success than was expected—are outcomes considered somewhat less likely to occur with treatment at the time of follow-up. The extreme levels on a guide—much less and much more than expected success—are outcomes considered unlikely to occur, yet still plausible given the circumstances. An examination of the suicide goal area for this woman reflects the outcome range thought appropriate for her. She was expected to have at least four suicidal impulses without acting on any. The much lower than expected success level designated for her was that she would commit suicide. The somewhat lower than expected success level for her was acting unsuccessfully on one suicidal impulse. The much higher than expected success level for her was reporting no suicidal impulses. The somewhat higher than expected success level for her is inferable from the adjacent outcome levels—reporting but not acting on one to three suicidal impluses.

Reviewing the Completed Follow-up Guide

This step is intended to determine errors in follow-up guide construction that may make follow-up scoring problematic. Common errors include:

1. Vagueness: Clear indicators of outcome must be provided.
2. Improper weighting: A follow-up guide with only some scales weighted cannot be scored. Either all or none of the scales must weighted.
3. Incompleteness: All five outcome levels must be complete or inferable in content.
4. Time-frame contradictions: Outcomes must all be geared to the same follow-up time interval.
5. Overlap: Outcome levels must be mutually exclusive or follow-up scoring is problematic.

6. Multiple dimensions in one scale: Scales should contain one behavioral dimension so that differential change among two or more dimensions does not confuse follow-up scoring.

Follow-up and the Goal Attainment Score

When the follow-up time interval has elapsed, an interview is typically held to determine which outcome levels on each scale best describe the client's status at that time. Often the information used to determine outcomes is asked within the context of a consumer satisfaction interview. In uses of GAS where the client has participated in guide construction, he or she often scores the guide or provides direct information for scoring. The follow-up outcome levels are usually determined by a mark such as an "x" or "*" on the guide itself. Each scale can be scored at only one level. The woman in Figure 7.5 attained one goal at the expected level, attained three goals at the somewhat more than expected level, and attained one goal at the much more than expected level.

The Goal Attainment Score can be calculated once follow-up has occurred and goal attainment for each scale has been indicated. The score may be considered to be an average of the outcome scores for all the goal areas on a follow-up guide, adjusted for the number of goals, the relative weights, and the typical intercorrelation among scales. Conceptually, the score is an index of the degree to which outcome expectations have been realized.

The formula to follow to derive the Goal Attainment Score (Kiresuk & Sherman, 1968) is displayed in Figure 7.6. At the time of follow-up, the levels of attainment (x_i) for each goal are determined. These levels, given values ranging from +2 to −2, and the relative goal weights (w_i), are used to generate a standardized score. This formula yields a single summary score for each follow-up guide that theoretically may range in distribution from 15 to 85. If outcomes are at the expected level, then the formula yields a score of 50 with a standard deviation of 10. This expected theoretical distribution is supported empirically. For example, in the original application of GAS at the Hennepin County Mental Health Service, 402 followed-up patients had a mean score of 51.9, with a standard deviation of 10.1. A distribution of these scores is represented in Figure 7.7.

Original Goal Attainment Score Formula:

$$Tj = 50 + \frac{10\Sigma w_j x_i}{\sqrt{(1 - p)\Sigma w_i^2 + p(\Sigma w_i)^2}}$$

where it is recommended that p be taken as about .30.

Modified Goal Attainment Formula:

$$T^1 = 50 + \frac{\Sigma w_j(T_j - 50)}{\sqrt{(7 - p)\Sigma w_j^2 + p(\Sigma w_j)^2}}$$

where it may be necessary to select a value for p commensurate with the intercorrelations of the sub-objective scores, T_j.

FIGURE 7.6. Original and modified goal attainment scaling formulas.

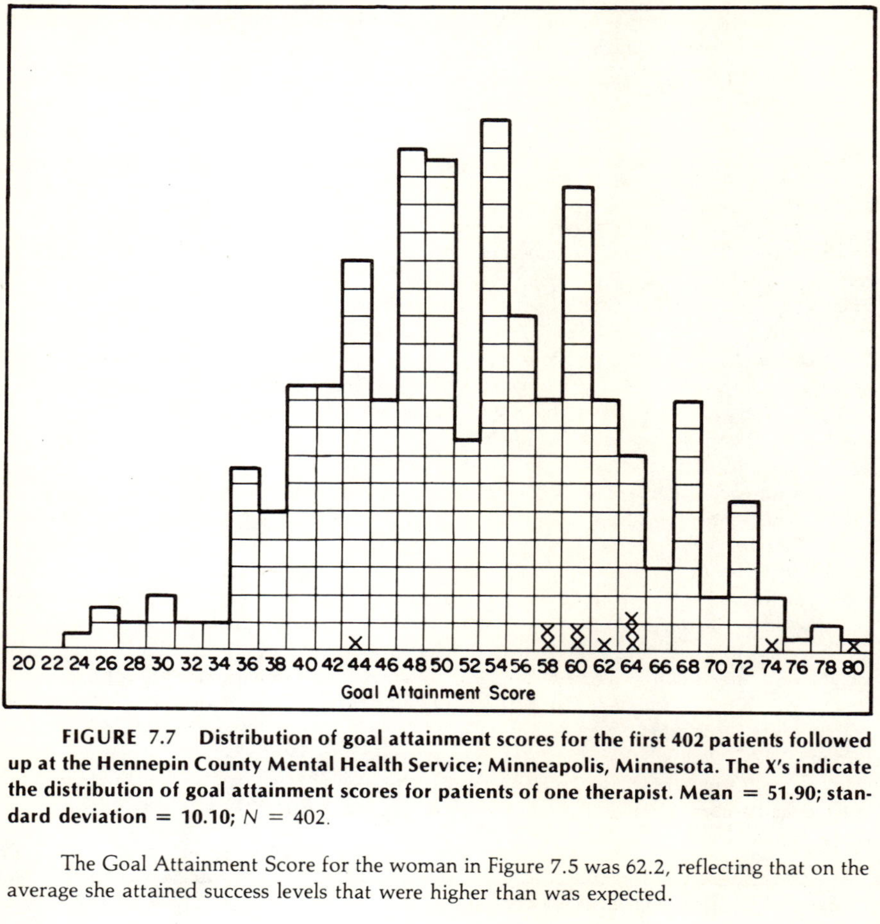

FIGURE 7.7 Distribution of goal attainment scores for the first 402 patients followed up at the Hennepin County Mental Health Service; Minneapolis, Minnesota. The X's indicate the distribution of goal attainment scores for patients of one therapist. Mean = 51.90; standard deviation = 10.10; *N* = 402.

The Goal Attainment Score for the woman in Figure 7.5 was 62.2, reflecting that on the average she attained success levels that were higher than was expected.

Reliability and Validity

Questions of the reliability and validity of the GAS has been considered elsewhere (Garwick, 1974; Sherman, Baxter, & Audette, 1974; Sherman, 1977). Of the many general sources of error variation or unreliability in test scores, two sources are particularly relevant to GAS. These are unreliability or inconsistency in construction of follow-up guides and unreliability in follow-up scoring of guides. A reliability study of 44 cases using two independent guide constructors and two independent follow-up scorers for each guide yielded an intraclass reliability estimate between .50 and .65, taking into account all major sources of variance. Computed separately, the reliability of follow-up scoring was estimated to be between .65 and .81 and the reliability of guide construction was estimated to .83 (Sherman *et al.*, 1974).

REFERENCES

Aslin, A. L. *Feminist and community mental health center psychologists' expectations of mental health for women.* Doctoral dissertation, University of Maryland, 1974, Dissertation Abstracts no. 75–11213.

Brodsky, A. M. Therapeutic aspects of consciousness-raising groups. In Rawlings, E.,& Carter, D. (Eds.), *Psychotherapy for women: Treatment toward equality.* Springfield, Ill.: Charles C Thomas, 1977.

Brodsky, A., Holroyd, J., Payton, C., Rubinstein, E., Rosenkrantz, P., Sherman, J., & Zell, F. Report of the task force on sex bias and sex-role stereotyping in psychotherapeutic practice. *American Psychologist,* 1975, *30,* 1169–1175.

Broverman, I. K., Broverman, D. M., Clarkson, F., Rosenkrantz, P. S., & Vogel, S. R. Sex role stereotypes and clinical judgments of mental health. *Journal of Consulting and Clinical Psychology,* 1970, *34,* 1–7.

Carlson, R. Understanding Women: Implications for personality theory and research. *Journal of Social Issues,* 1972, *28*(2), 17–33.

Chesler, P. *Women and madness.* New York: Doubleday, 1972.

Davis, H. R. A checklist for change. In National Institute of Mental Health, *A manual for research utilization,* Washington, D. C.: U.S. Government Printing Office, 1971.

Densen, P. Public accountability and reporting systems in medicare and other health programs. *New England Journal of Medicine,* 1973, *28,* 401–406.

Doherty, M. A. Sexual bias in personality theory. *The Counseling Psychologist,* 1973, *4*(1), 67–75.

Ellis, R. H., & Wilson, N. Goal-oriented automated progress note (GAP). *Four Ways to Goal Attainment, Evaluation* Special Monograph, 1, 1973.

Fabrikant, B. The psychotherapist and female patient: Perceptions, misperceptions, and change. In Franks, V., & Burtle, V. (Eds.), *Women in therapy: New psychotherapies for a changing society.* New York: Brunner/Mazel, 1974.

Feminist Counseling Collective. Feminist psychotherapy. *Social Policy,* 1975, *6,* 54–62.

Foundation for Health Care Evaluation, Professional Standards Review Organization for Minneapolis and St. Paul, Minnesota hospitals. Minneapolis, Minnesota, 1977.

Garwick, G. *An introduction to reliability and the goal attainment score.* Unpublished paper, Program Evaluation Resource Center, Minneapolis, Minnesota, 1974.

Glaser, E. M. Knowledge transfer and institutional change. *Professional Psychology,* 1973, *4,* 434–444.

Glaser, K. Women's self-help groups as an alternative to therapy. *Psychotherapy: Theory, Research, and Practice.* 1976, *13,* 77–81.

Havelock, R. G., & Lingwood, D. A. R & D utilization strategies and functions: An analytical comparison of four systems. Ann Arbor, Mich.: Institute for Social Research, University of Michigan, 1973.

Jakubowski, P. A. Self-assertion training procedures for women. In Rawlings E., & Carter, D. (Eds.), *Psychotherapy for women: Treatment toward equality.* Springfield, Ill.: Charles C Thomas, 1977.

Kiesler, D. J. Some myths of psychotherapy research and the search for a paradigm. *Psychological Bulletin,* 1966, *65,* 110–136.

Kiresuk, T. J., & Lund, S. H. Goal attainment scaling. In Attkisson, C. C., Hargreaves, W. A., & Horowitz, M. J. (Eds.), *Evaluation of human service programs.* New York: Academic Press, 1977.

Kiresuk, T. J., Lund, S. H., Schultz, S. K., & Larsen, N. E. Translating theory into practice:

Change research at the Program Evaluation Resource Center. *Evaluation*, 1977, *4*, 88–96.

Kiresuk, T. J., & Sherman, R. E. Goal attainment scaling: A general method of evaluating comprehensive community mental health programs. *Community Mental Health Journal*, 1968, *4*, 443–453.

Kirsh, B. Consciousness-raising groups as therapy for women. In Franks, V., & Burtle, V. (Eds.), *Women in therapy*. New York: Brunner/Mazel, 1974.

Klein, M. H. Feminist concepts of therapy outcome. *Psychotherapy: Theory, Research and Practice*. 1976, *13*, 89–95.

Kravetz, D. F. Consciousness-raising groups and group psychotherapy: Alternative mental health resources for women. *Psychotherapy: Theory, Research and Practice*. 1976, *13*, 66–71.

Mander, A. V., & Rush, A. K. *Feminism as therapy*. New York: Random House, 1974.

Maxfield, R. B. *Sex-role stereotypes of psychotherapists*. Doctoral dissertation, Adelphi University, New York, 1976, Dissertation Abstracts no. DAH 76–22816.

Orlinsky, D. E., & Howard, K. I. The effects of sex of therapist on the therapeutic experiences of women. *Psychotherapy: Theory, Research and Practice*, 1976, *13*, 82–88.

Rawlings, E. J., & Carter, D. K. *Psychotherapy for women: Treatment toward equality*. Springfield, Ill.: Charles C Thomas, 1977.

Sanders, C. J., & Stewart, D. C. Feminist bibliotherapy—prescription for change: A selected and annotated bibliotherapy. In Rawlings, E., & Carter, D. (Eds.), *Psychotherapy for women: Treatment toward equality*. Springfield, Ill.: Charles C Thomas, 1977.

Scriven, M. The methodology of evaluation. In Weiss, C. (Ed.), *Evaluating action programs: Readings in social action and education*. Boston: Allyn & Bacon, 1972.

Sherman, R. E. Will goal attainment scaling solve the problems of program evaluation in the mental health field? In *Program evaluation for mental health: Methods, strategies, and participants*, New York: Grune & Stratton, 1977.

Sherman, R. E., Baxter, J., & Audette, D. *An examination of the reliability of the Kiresuk-Sherman goal attainment score by means of components of variance*. Unpublished paper, Program Evaluation Project, 1974.

Sprei-Ott, J. *Feminist therapy: A review of the issues*. Unpublished paper, University of Maryland, Baltimore, 1976.

Stricker, G. Implications of research for psychotherapeutic treatment of women. *American Psychologist*, 1977, *32*, 14–22.

Thomas, S. A. Theory and practice in feminist therapy. *Social Work*, 1977, *22*(6), 447–455.

Walker, R., & Baxter, J. *Effects of clinical feedback*. Unpublished project report, Program Evaluation Resource Center, 1972.

Weed, L. L. *Medical records, medical examination and patient care*. Cleveland: Case Western Reserve University Press, 1969.

Woy, R. J., Lund, D. A., & Attkisson, C. C. Quality assurance in human service program evaluation. In Attkisson, C. C., Hargreaves, W. A., & Horowitz, M. J. (Eds.) *Evaluation of human service programs*. New York: Academic Press, 1978.

AFTERWORD

Deborah Belle
Susan Salasin

Despair, hopelessness, feelings of worthlessness, difficulty in sleeping and eating, loss of energy, and thoughts of death are some of the painful symptoms of depression. While women are not overrepresented in mental health facilities, they do suffer disproportionately from depression. The experts in this volume are agreed that the preponderance of women among those suffering from depression is real and not a product of medical misdiagnosis or incorrect self-labeling. Contrary to the widespread impression, depression today is not confined to women of late middle age. At every age, women are more likely than their male counterparts to experience depression.

The chapters in this volume have set out the facts and theories we have about depression, but they have arrived at no simple or definitive answers to many questions. Depression remains a puzzling illness, with probable multiple causes in social factors, loss and stress, biochemistry, heredity, learning history, and early socialization. It is of pressing importance that we solve the puzzle of depression so that we can more adequately treat and even prevent this problem.

From several pieces of evidence, we do know that depression is particularly likely to ensue when life presents exorbitant demands while offering few resources or options for coping with those demands. The impact of such demands, often called "stress," has been explored in this volume. What is surprising is that we know so little about the stresses of women's lives, and the impact of stress on women's mental health. Stress research has been dominated by studies of men, and the findings and theories developed from such studies have been improperly generalized to women. Yet there is evidence that women and men respond differently to the same stressful events.

Furthermore, stress research has concentrated on purely personal changes and has ignored societal changes, such as those in women's roles, which may be stressful. Although there is evidence that much of the stress in women's lives arises through "contagion," when events occur to other people important to the self and not to the self directly, few studies have investigated the stress experienced by women from events in the lives of their husbands or other persons close to them. Much stress in life is related not to how much things change but to how much an oppressive condition remains the same. This kind of stress has rarely been explored in research.

Such issues are urgent ones for the design and improvement of mental health services for women. While much therapy for women has been designed to help them adjust to existing social roles and demands, feminist therapy, which attributes women's pathology primarily to social and external rather than personal sources, can be a force for changing social roles. To the extent that depression results from oppressive social roles of women, such therapy could succeed when other types of therapy have failed in treating this mental health problem.

Since the stresses women experience are often generated in the broader social context, political action can advance the cause of women's well-being and mental health. To the extent that depression is a disease of powerlessness and hopelessness, political efforts to broaden women's options and their ability to control their own lives and improve their futures should aid the cause of women's mental health.

As this book goes to press, steps are being taken to build on this knowledge base and to translate the knowledge gained in this work into action on behalf of women. Susan Salasin and Deborah Belle are proceeding with the Stress and Families Project, focusing on the demographic group most at risk for depression—low-income mothers of young children. While not discounting the importance of other factors in the genesis of depression, the Stress and Families Project has emphasized the investigation of environmental risk factors. The project was designed to investigate the relationship between women's life situations and their mental health and to locate points at which interventions might be successful in protecting mental health and family functioning. Evidence from this new project will be relevant to the 4 million families and 10 million children living in poverty in this country today, as well as to other families living above the poverty line but suffering from financial strain.

To assure that the findings of the Stress and Families Project are translated into action on behalf of those victimized by their environment and those victimized by depression, the work of the project is aided by a National Advisory Committee. This distinguished group of mental health experts, researchers, policy experts, activists, and writers is chaired by Jeanette Williams of the U.S. Senate Committee on Human Resources. Building on the findings contained in this report, the National Advisory Committee will work with the research staff to develop specific policy recommendations and to recommend innovations in mental health services for women. In addition, the National Advisory Committee will work to mobilize the support necessary to turn these recommendations into reality. Their work helps to assure that the Stress and Families Project is truly a research-into-action project.

SUBJECT INDEX

PERSONALITY AND PSYCHOPATHOLOGY

A Series of Monographs, Texts, and Treatises

David T. Lykken, Editor

1. The Anatomy of Achievement Motivation, *Heinz Heckhausen.* 1966*
2. Cues, Decisions, and Diagnoses: A Systems-Analytic Approach to the Diagnosis of Psychopathology, *Peter E. Nathan.* 1967*
3. Human Adaptation and Its Failures, *Leslie Phillips.* 1968*
4. Schizophrenia: Research and Theory, *William E. Broen, Jr.* 1968*
5. Fears and Phobias, *I. M. Marks.* 1969
6. Language of Emotion, *Joel R. Davitz.* 1969
7. Feelings and Emotions, *Magda Arnold.* 1970
8. Rhythms of Dialogue, *Joseph Jaffe* and *Stanley Feldstein.* 1970
9. Character Structure and Impulsiveness, *David Kipnis.* 1971
10. The Control of Aggression and Violence: Cognitive and Physiological Factors, *Jerome L. Singer* (Ed.). 1971
11. The Attraction Paradigm, *Donn Byrne.* 1971
12. Objective Personality Assessment: Changing Perspectives, *James N. Butcher* (Ed.). 1972
13. Schizophrenia and Genetics, *Irving I. Gottesman* and *James Shields,* 1972*
14. Imagery and Daydream Methods in Psychotherapy and Behavior Modification, *Jerome L. Singer.* 1974
15. Experimental Approaches to Psychopathology, *Mitchell L. Kietzman, Samuel Sutton,* and *Joseph Zubin* (Eds.). 1975
16. Coping and Defending: Processes of Self-Environment Organization, *Norma Haan.* 1977
17. The Scientific Analysis of Personality and Motivation, *R. B. Cattell* and *P. Kline.* 1977
18. The Determinants of Free Will: A Psychological Analysis of Responsible, Adjustive Behavior, *James A. Easterbrook.*

*Titles initiated during the series editorship of Brendan Maher.

19. The Psychopath in Society, *Robert J. Smith.*

20. The Fears of Adolescents, *J. H. Bamber.*

21. Cognitive–Behavioral Interventions: Theory, Research, and Procedures, *Philip C. Kendall* and *Steven D. Hollon* (Eds.).

22. The Psychobiology of the Depressive Disorders: Implications for the Effects of Stress, *Richard A. Depue* (Ed.).

23. The Mental Health of Women, Marcia Guttentag, Susan Salasin, and Deborah Belle (Eds.).